Abderrezak Bouamra
Souad Meddah
Hanane Ammar Boudjellal

Hospital hygiene guide for healthcare staff

Abderrezak Bouamra
Souad Meddah
Hanane Ammar Boudjelal

Hospital hygiene guide for healthcare staff

Healthcare establishment

Imprint

Any brand names and product names mentioned in this book are subject to trademark, brand or patent protection and are trademarks or registered trademarks of their respective holders. The use of brand names, product names, common names, trade names, product descriptions etc. even without a particular marking in this work is in no way to be construed to mean that such names may be regarded as unrestricted in respect of trademark and brand protection legislation and could thus be used by anyone.

Cover image: www.ingimage.com

This book is a translation from the original published under ISBN 978-620-3-45364-5.

Publisher:
Sciencia Scripts
is a trademark of
Dodo Books Indian Ocean Ltd. and OmniScriptum S.R.L publishing group

120 High Road, East Finchley, London, N2 9ED, United Kingdom
Str. Armeneasca 28/1, office 1, Chisinau MD-2012, Republic of Moldova, Europe
Printed at: see last page
ISBN: 978-620-7-06294-2

Contents

CHAPTER I

General

I- HOSPITAL-ACQUIRED INFECTIONS

1. DEFINITION OF NOSOCOMIAL INFECTION

An infection is said to be nosocomial if it appears during or following hospitalisation and if it was not present on admission to hospital.

When the precise situation on admission is not known, a period of at least 48 hours after admission is commonly accepted to distinguish between a nosocomial and a community-acquired infection.

For surgical site infections, infections occurring within 30 days of the operation or, if a prosthesis or implant has been fitted, within one year of the operation, are considered to be nosocomial.

2. SCOPE OF THE PROBLEM

Nosocomial infections are responsible for a high level of morbidity and mortality in healthcare establishments. According to various studies carried out in hospitals in developed countries, 5 to 10% of hospitalised patients acquire a nosocomial infection.

According to the various surveys of the prevalence of nosocomial infection carried out in Algeria across the different hospital establishments. The instantaneous prevalence varied between 3.9% and 15.2%.

3. CIRCUMSTANCES FAVOURING THE OCCURRENCE OF A NOSOCOMIAL INFECTION

Among the situations that can be implicated in the transmission of nosocomial infections, the most important are :

- ill-suited architecture ;
- overcrowding, overcrowding, overcrowded services;
- failure to maintain and disinfect the premises ;
- misuse of hospital hygiene products ;
- the lack of isolation of patients who are infected or at risk of infection;
- non-compliance with food, linen and healthcare waste circuits;
- the lack of personal hygiene among patients and staff;
- inadequate hand washing and disinfection ;
- non-rigorous care gestures ;
- environmental contamination (air, water, etc.);
- poor work organisation;
- Therapeutic pressure (antibiotics, corticoids, etc.);
- non-compliance with protocols and procedures.

4. RECEPTIVE SUBJECTS

All patients are more or less immunocompromised and therefore susceptible to infection following hospital contamination. Staff are very often exposed to contamination, but rarely fall victim to infection.

Particularly receptive:

- immunocompromised patients, primary or secondary to treatment (cancer, AIDS, etc.);
- patients with damaged skin (burns, bedsores, polytrauma, etc.);
- diabetics ;
- respiratory insufficiency;
- kidney failure ;
- people with dementia, who often have several illnesses at the same time;
- newborn babies, especially premature ones, with immature immune systems;
- subjects with risk factors for disease (smokers, alcoholics, etc.).

5. SERVICES AT RISK

The risk of nosocomial infection is linked either to the state of health of patients admitted to the department, or to the therapies and/or invasive procedures carried out there, or to both these factors at the same time.

Services at risk include :

- intensive care units :
- surgery and neurosurgery departments,
- neonatology department,
- catheter and pacemaker implantation service

6. MODES OF TRANSMISSION

There are two types of infection linked to the different reservoirs:

Endogenous infection: infection acquired from the patient's own germs (skin, mucous membrane, digestive tract), sometimes facilitated by the surgical procedure, a leaking suture, care, etc.

Exogenous infection: by far the most important, acquired from the patient's environment. A distinction is made between :

- cross infections, often carried by staff, are the most common infections;
- infections caused by germs from outside the hospital, imported by patients, visitors and staff,
- infections caused by germs imported by accident (polluted water, defective sterilisation, unfiltered air, air conditioning, etc.);
- collective food poisoning.

7. THE GERMS RESPONSIBLE

At present, the most frequently identified micro-organisms are : Escherichia coli and other enterobacteria, Staphylococcus aureus, Pseudomonas aeruginosa, klebsiella, acetobacter Baumannii.

The main micro-organisms responsible for nosocomial infections, their main reservoir and their mode of transmission are described in the table below.

MICRO-ORGANISMS RESPONSIBLE FOR NOSOCOMIAL INFECTIONS, THEIR MAIN RESERVOIR, MODE OF TRANSMISSION AND MAIN ROUTE OF ENTRY

Micro-organism	Species	Main tank	Transmission mode	Main entrance door
GRAM-POSITIVE COCCI				
Staphylococcus	Epidermidis Aureus	Human and animal Skin and mucous membranes Environment Human Nasopharynx and skin Environment	Direct contact Indirect contact including manu portage Direct contact Indirect contact including manu portage	Percutaneous mucocutaneous Mucocutaneous Percutaneous Digestive Respiratory
Streptococcus	A, B, C...	Human	Direct contact Droplets Indirect contact including manu portage	Mucocutaneous Digestive Respiratory Maternal-fetal
Enterococcus	D	Human and animal Digestive tract Environment	Indirect contact including manu portage	Digestive
GRAM-POSITIVE BACILLI				
Bacillus	Cereus	Environment : soil germ	Direct contact	Digestive
Listeria	Monocytogenes	Environment	Direct contact: rare Indirect contact	Digestive Respiratory Maternal-fetal
ACID-FAST BACILLI				
Mycobacterium	Tuberculosis	Human: respiratory	Aeroporte: droplets	Respiratory

Micro-organism	Species	Main tank	Transmission mode	Main entrance door
MUSHROOMS				
Candida	Albicans	Human Animal Environment	Direct contact Indirect contact including manu portage	Digestive
Aspergillus	Fumigatus	Environment: vegetation, decomposing organic matter, soil, dust	Aeroporte	Respiratory
GRAM-NEGATIVE BACILLI				
Acinetobacter	Baumanii	Human: skin and mucous membranes	Indirect contact including manu portage	Mucocutaneous Digestive
Escherichia	Coli	Human and animal: digestive tract	Indirect contact including manu portage	Digestive
Klebsiella	Pneumoniae	Human and animal: digestive tract Environment: soil, water, plants	Indirect contact including manu portage	Mucocutaneous Digestive Respiratory
Enterobacter		Human and animal: digestive tract	Direct contact Indirect contact including	Mucocutaneous Digestive Respiratory

Micro-organism	Species	Main tank	Transmission mode	Main entrance door
		Environment: soil, water, manu portage plants		
Serratia	Marcescens	Human and animal: digestive tract Environment: soil, water, manu portage plants	Indirect contact including manu portage	Mucocutaneous Digestive
Proteus		Human and animal: digestive tract	Indirect contact including manu portage	Digestive
Legionella		Environment: especially water	Aeroportee: droplets	Respiratory
Pseudomonas	Aeruginosa	Human and animal: digestive tract Environment: soil, water, plants	Indirect contact including manu portage	Mucocutaneous Digestive Respiratory
Micro-organism	**Species**	**Main tank**	**Transmission mode**	**Main entrance door**
STRICT ANAEROBIC SPOROGENIC BACTERIA				
Clostridium	Difficult	Human Animal Environment	Indirect contact including manu portage	Digestive
	Perfringens	Human Animal Environment	Indirect contact including manu portage	Mucocutaneous Percutaneous Digestive
	Tetani	Animal Environment: soil, water	Indirect contact	Mucocutaneous Percutaneous
VIRUS				
Hepatitis viruses	A	Human	Indirect contact including manu portage	Digestive
	B	Human	Direct contact: rare Indirect contact	Percutaneous Sexual Maternal-fetal Blood
	C	Human	Direct contact Indirect contact	Percutaneous Sexual Maternal-fetal Blood
HIV		Human	Direct contact Indirect contact	Percutaneous Sexual Maternal-fetal Blood

II- SURVEILLANCE OF NOSOCOMIAL INFECTIONS

1. DEFINITION AND OBJECTIVES OF NOSOCOMIAL INFECTION SURVEILLANCE

Monitoring is the process of collecting, compiling and analysing data, and disseminating it to all those who need to know.

Surveillance of hospital-acquired infections is an essential activity because it provides the epidemiological information that is essential for :

• measuring the level of infectious risks in a risk department or healthcare establishment ;

• defining the prevention policy to be implemented ;

• evaluating the effectiveness of this prevention policy: surveillance data can be used as an indicator to measure the impact of a prevention programme.

2. MONITORING METHODS

It is important to use standardised monitoring methods that can produce comparable data over time and space.

There are several stages in the surveillance of nosocomial infections:

• identifying patients who have contracted a nosocomial infection;

• the collection of relevant epidemiological information (particularly concerning the distribution of the main risk factors) on all patients under surveillance: infected and non-infected patients;

• calculating and analysing infection rates ;

• finally, rapid feedback to the medical and paramedical teams concerned, so that appropriate control and prevention measures can be put in place.

Surveillance is an active process: information is collected systematically by staff who have received appropriate training.

Two types of study can be used to monitor nosocomial infections: cross-sectional studies and cohort studies.

1.1.Cross-sectional study (or prevalence survey) :

It is based on the monitoring of all patients hospitalised at a given time in the department(s) being monitored. Each patient's infection status is assessed only once. At the end of the study, an instantaneous prevalence is calculated. This method can be used at regular intervals, for example every year at the same time.

This type of study, which is easy to carry out thanks to its limited duration, provides an initial assessment of the extent of infectious risks and, if repeated, enables us to monitor trends in these risks over time.

1.2.Cohort studies (or incidence studies) :

It is based on continuous monitoring of a group of patients over time, with recording of new cases of infection occurring during hospitalisation and after the patient has been discharged (particularly in surgery). Each patient's infection status is assessed for the entire hospital stay. At the end of the study, an incidence density and/or attack rate is calculated.

This type of study makes it possible to accurately determine the rates of nosocomial infections and to identify the major infectious risk factors. During the course of this type of surveillance, it is possible to detect any epidemic of nosocomial infections as soon as it emerges, provided that the follow-up period is long and the surveillance data are analysed regularly.

3. TARGET SERVICES

All the departments of a hospital establishment with an inpatient activity may be subject to surveillance for nosocomial infections.

In the case of cross-functional studies, it is advisable to include all the departments of the establishment concerned, or better still, all the departments of the establishments in the region.

In cohort studies, it would be preferable to target only those departments at high risk of nosocomial infection in the institution concerned, i.e. surgery, intensive care, resuscitation, neonatology and onco-hematology departments.

4. DEFINITIONS USED TO IDENTIFY NOSOCOMIAL INFECTIONS

Standardised definitions of nosocomial infections with criteria corresponding to each anatomical location have been proposed by the Centers for Disease Control and Prevention (1988, 1992, 1995). However, because of their simplicity, in this manual we will only present the definitions of the French National Technical Committee on nosocomial infections for the 05 most frequent sites.

4.1.Surgical site infection

Infections occurring within 30 days of the operation or, if a prosthesis or implant has been fitted, within one year of the operation, are considered to be nosocomial. Depending on the location in relation to the incision, a distinction is made between 03 types of infection: superficial infection of the incision, deep infection of the incision and infection of the organ, site or space.

4.1.1. Superficial infection of the incision

Infection occurring within 30 days of the operation and affecting the skin (or mucous membranes), subcutaneous tissue or tissue above the covering aponeurosis, diagnosed by :

Case 1: Purulent or puriform discharge from the incision or drain.

Case 2: Micro-organism isolated by culture from the fluid produced by a closed wound or tissue sample.

Case 3: Opening by the surgeon in the presence of any of the following signs: pain or tenderness on palpation, local tumour, redness, warmth (unless the culture of the wound sample is negative).

Case 4: Diagnosis of infection by the surgeon or doctor.

4.1.2. Deep infection of the incision

Infection occurring within 30 days of the operation, or within one year if an implant or prosthesis has been inserted, affecting tissues or spaces at or below the aponeurosis covering, diagnosed by :

Case 1: Purulent or puriform discharge from a sub-aponeurotic drain.

Case 2: Presence of one of the following signs:

- spontaneous dehiscence of the incision, scar or wall ;
- opening by the surgeon in the event of fever $> 38°C$, local pain, tenderness to palpation (unless the wound sample is culture negative).

Case 3: Abcesses or other signs of infection observed during reintervention or histopathological examination.

Case 4: Diagnosis of infection by the surgeon or doctor.

4.1.3. Organ or space infection

Infection occurring within 30 days of the operation, or within one year if an implant or prosthesis has been inserted, involving organs or spaces (other than the incision) opened or manipulated during the operation, diagnosed by:

Case 1: Presence of frank pus or puriform liquid from a drain placed in the organ, site or space.

Case 2: Micro-organism isolated by culture from an organ, site or space sample.

Case 3: Clear signs of infection involving the organ, site or space, observed during reintervention surgery or histopathological examination.

Case 4: Diagnosis of infection by the surgeon or doctor.

4.2. Urinary tract infection

4.2.1. Asymptomatic bacteriuria

Case 1: A positive quantitative uroculture (^{3} 105 micro-organisms/millilitre), if the patient has been catheterised in the week preceding the sample.

Case 2: In the absence of sampling, two consecutive positive quantitative urocultures (3,105 micro-organisms/millilitre) with the same micro-organism(s) with no more than two isolated micro-organisms.

4.2.2. Symptomatic bacteriuria (in patients with or without catheters)

- Fever ($> 38°C$) with no other infectious site and/or urge to urinate and/or dysuria and/or pollakiuria and/or suprapubic pressure
- AND a positive uroculture (^{3} 105 micro-organisms/millilitre) with no more

than two isolated microbial species, or a positive uroculture (3 10^3 micro-organisms/millilitre) with leucocyturia (3 104 leucocytes/millilitre).

4.3. Infectious lung disease

Radiological diagnosis (chest X-ray, CT scan) of one or more abnormal, recent and progressive parenchymal opacities.

AND one of the following characteristics:

Case 1: **identification of an isolated micro-organism :**
- sputum if it is a pathogenic micro-organism that is never commensal in the bronchi: Legionella pneumophila, Aspergillus fumigatus, mycobacteria, respiratory syncitial virus, etc;
- or, bronchoalveolar lavage with at least 5% of cells containing micro-organisms on direct microscopic examination after appropriate centrifugation, or more than 104 micro-organisms/millilitre;
- or, a protected telescopic brush sampling or a protected distal tracheal catheter sampling with more than10 micro^3
organisms/millilitre (in the absence of recently instituted antibiotic therapy) ;
- or a puncture of a pulmonary or levator abscess;
- or infectious pneumonitis or an abcess authenticated by histological examination.

Case 2: **a serodiagnosis, if the antibody level is considered significant by the laboratory** (e.g. *Legionella*).

Case 3: **at least one of the following signs:**
- purulent sputum (or tracheal secretion in ventilated patients) of recent onset ;
- fever higher than 38.5°C of recent onset in the absence of other causes;
- blood culture positive for a pathogenic micro-organism in the absence of any other outbreak and after ruling out a catheter infection.

4.4. Bacteria

At least one positive blood culture taken at peak temperature (with or without other clinical signs), **except for** the following micro-organisms:
- Coagulase-negative staphylococci;
- Bacillus spp;
- Corynebacterium spp. ;
- Propionibacterium spp;
- Micrococcus spp;
- or other saprophytic or commensal micro-organisms with comparable pathogenic potential;

for which two positive blood cultures taken from different punctures at different times are required.

4.5.Catheter infection

4.5.1. Local infection

Frank pus or puriform liquid at the catheter exit point or tunnelling.

4.5.2. Catheter infection with bacteremia

Positive peripheral blood culture (taken by venipuncture)

AND one of the following criteria:

Case 1: Local infection AND isolation of the same micro-organism in pus and peripheral blood.

Case 2: Positive catheter culture (Brun-Buisson quantitative method: > 1000 CFU/millilitre or Maki semi-quantitative method: > 15 CFU/millilitre, AND isolation of the same micro-organism as in the blood culture.

Case 3: The ratio of the concentration of micro-organisms (CFU/millilitre) in the blood culture taken from the catheter to the concentration of micro-organisms (CFU/millilitre) in the peripheral blood culture(s) > 5.

᾿ CFU: Colony forming unit

Case 4: Clinical signs of infection resistant to antibiotic therapy but disappearing 48 hours after catheter removal.

Case 5: Clinical signs of infection when handling the catheter.

5. METHODS FOR CALCULATING NOSOCOMIAL INFECTION RATES

5.1.Instant prevalence

Instantaneous prevalence is a proportion calculated by dividing the number of infected patients (or infections) on a given day (numerator) by the number of patients present on that day (denominator). The situation of each patient is examined at a single point in time.

Prévalence des patients infectés (ou des infections nosocomiales)	=	$\dfrac{\text{Nombre de patients infectés (ou d'infections) un jour donné}}{\text{Nombre de patients hospitalisés présents le même jour}}$	x100

Patient prevalence infected (or infections nosocomial)	$\dfrac{\text{Number of infected patients (or infections) one given day}}{\text{Number of inpatients present on the same day}}$

The instantaneous prevalence of infection is expressed per 100 hospitalised patients.

5.2.Incidence density

Incidence density is calculated by dividing the number of newly infected patients (or new cases of infection) occurring during a given period (numerator) by the total length of time patients were exposed to the risk during this same period (denominator). The duration of exposure to risk for a patient is evaluated, depending on the case, until discharge, death, or the end of the observation period for a non-infected patient, and until the date of onset of the nosocomial infection for infected patients.

The duration of exposure to a specific risk can be used to calculate incidence densities for specific infections.

$$\text{Densité d'incidence des patients infectés (ou des infections nosocomiales)} = \frac{\text{Nombre de patients nouvellement infectés (ou de cas d'infections) durant une période déterminé}}{\text{Total des durées d'hospitalisation à risque des patients durant la même période}} \times 1000$$

$$\text{Incidence density of infected patients (or nosocomial infections)} = \frac{\text{Number of newly infected patients (or of infections during a given period}}{\text{Total length of hospitalisation at risk for patients during the same period}}$$

The incidence density is expressed per 1000 days of hospitalisation or exposure to a specific risk.

5.3. Attack rate (or cumulative incidence)

The attack rate is calculated by dividing the number of newly infected patients (or new cases of infection) occurring during a given period (numerator) by the total number of patients hospitalised at risk during the same period (denominator), and expresses the risk of a patient contracting an infection per unit of time. These patients must be monitored throughout their hospital stay. Specific attack rates can be calculated by relating the number of patients with a specific infection (or the number of new cases of the infection concerned) to the number of patients exposed to the specific risk.

$$\text{Taux d'attaque des patients infectés (ou des infections nosocomiales)} = \frac{\text{Nombre de patients nouvellement infectés (ou de cas d'infections) durant une période déterminé}}{\text{Nombre de patients à risque hospitalisés durant la même période et suivies jusqu'à leur sortie}} \times 100$$

Attack rate of infected patients (or nosocomial infections)

$$\frac{\text{Number of newly infected patients (or cases of infection) during a given period}}{\text{Number of at-risk patients hospitalised during the same period and monitored until discharge}} \times 100$$

The attack rate is expressed per 100 patients hospitalised or exposed to the specific risk.

6. SURVEILLANCE STRATEGY FOR NOSOCOMIAL INFECTIONS

Each hospital establishes its own strategy for monitoring nosocomial infections, taking account of these priorities and its material and human resources.

The following table shows the main monitoring programmes and their constraints.

NOSOCOMIAL INFECTION SURVEILLANCE PROGRAMMES

Nature of surveillance	Services concerned	Infections monitored	Frequency of collection	Collection points	Minimum information to be collected	Determined indicators
Prevalence survey	All hospital departments	Urinary tract infections Infectious lung diseases Bacteremia Catheter infections Surgical site infections	One day gives	Clinical Department, Central Laboratory	Administrative data Number of patients present, Infectious site, Micro-organisms responsible	Instant prevalence
Impact survey	Surgical departments Intensive care units	Surgical site infections Urinary tract infections, Infectious lung diseases Bacteremia Catheter infections	03 months per year Continue	Operating theatre, Surgical resuscitation Surgical consultations Central laboratory Clinical department Central laboratory	Administrative data, operating risk factors, infectious site, micro-organisms responsible Administrative data Patient-related risk factors, Invasive manoeuvres Infectious site Micro-organisms responsible	Attack rate Incidence density

ORGANISATION OF THE FIGHT AGAINST NOSOCOMIAL INFECTIONS IN ALGERIA

The fight against hospital-acquired infections is still in its infancy in Algeria. The National Hospital Hygiene Committee was set up in March 1998. In November 1998, a ministerial decree set up a nosocomial infection control committee (CLIN) in each health establishment.

The CLIN is the official body within the health establishment responsible for organising the fight against nosocomial infections. It is an advisory body responsible for :

1. identify and monitor nosocomial infections and determine their frequency;

2. drawing up and proposing a programme to combat nosocomial infections and a training programme;

3. evaluate the results of actions undertaken and report back to the head of the school.

The role of the CLIN is to organise, plan and lead the fight against nosocomial infections in the hospital, in close collaboration with the hospital director, the medical and paramedical staff, and anyone involved in any way in promoting hospital hygiene. It defines the policy to be implemented by the hospital hygiene team and all the medical, paramedical and technical staff in the departments.

In addition to the CLIN, hospital hygiene units have been set up in the epidemiology and preventive medicine departments of university hospitals and health sectors. These units monitor hospital-acquired infections and evaluate hospital hygiene techniques. Training in hospital hygiene is regularly provided by these units for the establishment's medical, paramedical and technical staff.

III- PREREQUISITES FOR HOSPITAL HYGIENE

1. INTRODUCTION

The basic hygiene rules apply to patients and all medical and paramedical staff in the establishment. Their aim is to limit the risk of cross-transmission of micro-organisms responsible for nosocomial infections. Among the preventive measures, we will initially focus on body hygiene and clothing, which we consider to be the prerequisites for any other hospital hygiene action.

2. BODY HYGIENE

A daily shower is necessary before starting work in order to reduce the microbial flora. It is preferable to take this shower on the ward, but if this is not possible, it can be taken at home before leaving for work. Body linen is changed after the shower. Hair is kept clean and short. If hair is long, it should be tied back.

Jewellery is not permitted: no rings, watches, bracelets, dangling earrings or long necklaces. Wedding rings may be worn if they are smooth.

Nails must be clean, short and free of varnish.

Washing your hands is always a good idea before getting out of bed and after removing your work clothes.

3. PROFESSIONAL ATTIRE

The purpose of hospital workwear is to replace street clothes in order to limit the risk of infection from micro-organisms, thereby protecting patients and nursing staff.

The basic outfit will therefore have to comply with rules on form, material and maintenance.

3.1. The basic outfit

The basic professional outfit consists of :

- a blouse or tunic and trousers; the blouse or tunic must be short-sleeved;
- shoes designed for work, quiet and easy to care for. It is recommended that these shoes be closed at the top for safety and at the back for ergonomics.

Pockets should be straight and flat to avoid snagging and unnecessary overloading.

Fastenings should be without conventional buttonholes or cuffs to prevent dust accumulation. Press studs are preferred for fastening.

The colours must be different for different categories of personnel.

In terms of textiles, the polyester-cotton blend (65%-35%) is the benchmark for hospital staff clothing.

Professional clothing is worn exclusively on the premises of the establishment by anyone providing or observing care: professionals, students and trainees.

Personal items (scarves, waistcoats, etc.) are not permitted during treatment or in high-risk areas. A personal short-sleeved T-shirt is permitted under the uniform.

The watch must be specific to the job, attached to the tunic or blouse and easy to clean.

Professional clothing is changed daily and whenever necessary (in the event of soiling).

Professional clothing is always removed on leaving the service.

3.2. Specific clothing depending on the risk of contamination

3.2.1. Low-risk sectors

The services concerned are medical care, surgical care, outpatient care, consultations and radiology.

The recommended outfit is the basic one.

3.2.2. Moderate risk areas

The departments concerned are the intensive care unit, the intensive care unit and the operating theatre (excluding the peri-operative area).

Depending on the department, certain items may need to be worn: masks for respiratory isolation, over-gowns if there is a risk of contact with soiled patients or patients with a high risk of contamination.

The elements of the outfit are as follows:

- basic clothing ;
- a protective gown or single-use apron;
- sector-specific footwear.

The headdress and mask are not compulsory.

The mid-calf overblouse must be pocketless and short-sleeved.

The tunic and trousers must have no pockets, collars, lapels or buttons.

If a cap is used, it should be wraparound and light (like a nonwoven charlotte), and the surgical mask should cover the nose, mouth and chin.

The uniform must be changed daily and whenever it is soiled. The gown is changed at each shift change. The mask is put on at the entrance to the room and removed as soon as the patient leaves. It is effective for a maximum of 3 hours.

The overblouse must be hung on a coat rack inside the room. It should be hung on the outside to limit the risk of contamination.

3.2.3. High-risk sectors

The departments concerned are operating theatres in the perioperative area, interventional radiology, and wards where immunodeficient patients are hospitalised (in protective isolation).

People carrying out aseptic procedures (insertion of central catheter, cardiac training probe, etc.) are also required to wear this outfit.

The elements of the outfit are :

- a tunic and trousers;
- a sterile surgical gown;
- a sterile cap and mask, preferably disposable;
- single-use sterile gloves;
- specific footwear.

The tunic, with short sleeves and no pockets, cuffs, waistband or buttons, must be tucked into the trousers to avoid the shirt effect. The bottom of the trousers must be tight.

The sterile surgical gown must have long sleeves, tight at the wrists and covering the ankles.

The headdress should be as full-covering as possible (no fringe on the forehead), like a nonwoven charlotte.

The surgical mask must cover the nose, mouth and chin.

The surgical gown must be changed for each operation, the tunic and trousers must be changed daily, the cap and gloves must be changed for each operation, and the mask must be changed every 3 hours and for each operation.

The uniforms must be removed on leaving the block or unit and replaced with basic clothing.

IV- HAND HYGIENE

1. INTRODUCTION AND DEFINITIONS

More than 90% of hospital-acquired infections are carried directly or indirectly. Hand washing is the best way of preventing hospital-acquired infections. Its aim is to reduce the microbial flora present on the surface of the skin, and so prevent the transmission of micro-organisms from one patient to another.

It is therefore essential to promote hand washing by healthcare staff, but this can only be done properly if there are enough water points on the ward and they are properly equipped.

The skin flora is made up of two types of micro-organisms:

• **The** skin's **commensal bacteria** are permanently and habitually present. These bacteria make up the resident flora. This flora plays an important barrier role, preventing colonisation by other species.

• **Saprophytic bacteria live** briefly on the skin and come from the environment. These bacteria make up the transient flora. This flora is mainly responsible for cross-infections.

2. STEPS AND OBJECTIVES OF HAND WASHING

Steps	Objectives
Soaping	Produce foam that envelops micro-organisms on the surface of the skin
Ringage	- Eliminate foam and micro-organisms using the mechanical action of water - Eliminate soap and protect the skin surface
Drying	- To prevent the skin from drying out - Avoiding microbial proliferation due to excess humidity

3. PRODUCTS REQUIRED

As bar soap is banned because it encourages the transmission of germs, liquid soap, the type of which varies depending on the type of handwashing to be carried out, and hydro-alcoholic solutions are used for handwashing.

Hydroalcoholic solution is a quick-drying solution for hand antisepsis, containing one or more antiseptic agents, including alcohol, and one or more skin-protecting emollients.

The different liquid soaps and hydroalcoholic solutions available, along with their action and indications, are shown in the table below.

Liquid soapActionIndications	Availability
GentleDetergentSingle wash	Commercially available.
Detergent and washing Д nticpnti лир rmlseULUUe hygienic antiseptic	CHLORIDERM® is marketed by ANIOS/NOSOCLEAN Laboratories (194, rue Boudjemaa Khelil, Oued Romane, 16403 El-Achour, Algiers).

Chimruic,! ^{Deter}gente ^{and} Washing ^{Chi}IUI^{gical} surgical antiseptic	DERMANIOS SCRUB HF® marketed by ANIOS/NOSOCLEAN laboratories; BETADINE SCRUB® marketed by ASTA MEDICA laboratories.
SolutionsSimple washing, hydro-Antiseptic hygienic and surgical	MANUGEL® marketed by ANIOS/NOSOCLEAN laboratories.

4. MATERIAL REQUIRED

- Equipped water point: deep washbasin, without overflow if possible, with unobstructed taps;
- Liquid soap dispenser that can be operated by the elbow (alternatively a measuring bottle can be used);
- Hand towel dispenser ;
- Single-use hand towels ;
- Manual contactless waste collector: pedal bin.

For surgical scrubbing :

- Taps should be hand-free;
- Hand towels must be sterile;
- Sterile, single-use nail brushes.

5. THE DIFFERENT TYPES OF HAND WASHING

5.1. Simple washing

5.1.1. Objectives

Eliminate dirt and reduce transient flora by simple mechanical action.

5.1.2. Equipment and products required

- Mild liquid soap ;
- Water from the network ;
- Non-sterile single-use hand towels.

5.1.3. Indications

This is the type of wash to be used after any routine procedure, and before and after any procedure with a low level of infectious risk:

- on arrival and departure ;
- before and after any contact with a patient ;
- between two activities ;
- after having combed their hair;
- after going to the toilet;
- before and after smoking;
- before and after meals;
- before and after wearing non-sterile gloves...

5.1.4. Technical

- Denuder hands and forearms;
- Wet hands and wrists;
- Take a dose of liquid soap;
- Lather thoroughly for at least 15 seconds, paying particular attention to the interdigital spaces, nail edges, palms, wrists and ulnar edges;
- Rinse thoroughly, lifting your hands so that the rinse water flows towards your wrists;
- Pat dry with a single-use hand towel;
- Close the tap without touching it, possibly with the last towel used if the control is manual;
- Throw away the towel without touching the bin.

The minimum wash time is 30 seconds.

5.2. Hygienic washing

5.2.1. Objectives

Remove dirt and eliminate or reduce **transient flora** by mechanical action and the action of antiseptic soap.

5.2.2. Equipment and products required

- Liquid antiseptic soap ;
- Water from the network ;
- Non-sterile single-use hand towels.

5.2.3. Indications

This type of washing is carried out before any procedure with an intermediate level of infectious risk:

- before carrying out an invasive procedure: inserting a peripheral venous line, catheters, urinary catheter, dressing, drain care, etc.
- for handling sterile materials ;
- before any contact with immunocompromised patients;
- after any contact with infected patients or patients in septic isolation;
- if multi-resistant bacteria are present ;
- in the event of contact with blood, biological fluids or organic materials;
- before wearing sterile gloves...

5.2.4. Technical

- Denuder hands and forearms;
- Wet hands and wrists;
- Take a dose of antiseptic liquid soap;
- Soap thoroughly for at least 30 to 60 seconds, not forgetting the fingertips, interdigital spaces and the tops of the wrists;
- Rinse thoroughly, lifting your hands so that the ringing water flows towards

your wrists;
- Pat dry with the hand towel;
- Close the tap without touching it, possibly using a hand towel if the control is manual;
- Throw away the towel without touching the bin.

Minimum soaping time: 30 to 60 seconds = time needed for the antiseptic contained in the soap to take effect.

5.3.Surgical lavage

5.3.1. Objectives

Remove dirt, eliminate **transient flora and reduce** long-lasting **flora** by mechanical action and the action of antiseptic soap.

5.3.2. Equipment and products required
- Major liquid antiseptic soap ;
- Sterile single-use nail brush;
- Bacteriologically controlled water (faulty, mains water) ;
- Single-use sterile (or non-sterile) hand towels.

5.3.3. Indications

This is the type of wash that should be carried out for any procedure involving a high level of infectious risk:
- Before any surgical, obstetric or interventional radiology procedure;
- Before any procedure requiring rigorous asepsis (insertion of a central catheter, spinal catheter, implantable chamber, amniotic puncture, insertion of a chest tube, etc.).

5.3.4. Technical

The procedure lasts at least 05 minutes, divided into three stages.

1ᵉᵉ time: Prewash
- Wear a mask and a cap covering the hair;
- Bare hands and forearms above the elbows;
- Get your hands and forearms wet;
- Apply a dose of soap and massage into a rich lather from fingertips to elbows for one (01) minute/second = two (02) minutes in total;
- Keep your hands above your elbows throughout the operation;
- Rinse thoroughly.

2ᵉᵐᵉ time:
- Take another dose of soap;
- Massage into a lather using the same technique;
- Take a sterile brush;
- Brush the nails and count 30 seconds per hand = one (01) minute in total;
- Keep your hands above your elbows throughout the operation;

*   Rinse thoroughly.

3^{ëme} time:

*   Take another dose of soap, massage for one (01) minute (hands, wrists and forearms) then rinse;
*   Dab dry with a single-use hand towel (preferably sterile), one per limb, moving from the hands to the elbow;
*   Hold your hand up;
*   Maintain the same position when dressing;
*   one (01) minute per hand, 30 seconds per forearm = three (03) minutes in total.

5.4. Hygienic hand treatment by friction

5.4.1. Objectives

This treatment replaces simple hand washing and hygienic hand washing.

5.4.2. Equipment and products required

- Hydroalcoholic solution.

5.4.3. Indications

The instructions are identical to those for simple washing and hygienic washing. Do not rub your hands, but wash them if they are dirty, damp, powdery, chalky or smeared.

The use of these solutions is recommended because they are very well tolerated and lead to better compliance with hand washing.

5.4.4. Technical

*   Denuder hands and forearms;
*   Take a dose of hydro-alcoholic solution;
*   Rub your hands for 30 to 60 seconds: palm, back, interdigital spaces, ulnar edge, until the skin is completely dry.

5.5. Surgical hand disinfection by friction

5.5.1. Objectives

This treatment replaces surgical hand washing.

5.5.2. Equipment and products required

*   Mild liquid soap ;
*   Water from the network ;
*   Single-use non-sterile nail brush;
*   Single-use non-sterile towels;
*   Hydroalcoholic solution.

5.5.3. Indications

The indications are identical to those for surgical hand washing. This technique is highly recommended for its simplicity. No special equipment is required, the water used is mains water, and the nail brush and hand towel used are non-sterile.

5.5.4. Technical

- Denuder hands and forearms above the elbows;
- Start by washing your hands and forearms (including elbows);
- Brush your nails for 01 minute (30 seconds per hand);
- Rinse ;
- Dry hands thoroughly with single-use non-sterile towels;
- 1ere hand rubbing up to and including elbows, until completely dry (time > 01 minute);
- 2eme rubbing from hands to forearms (elbows excluded), until completely dry (time > 01 minute).

6. EVALUATION OF HAND WASHING

Assessment is carried out by means of audits. An audit may be organised periodically by the medical supervisor or the hospital's hygiene department. The periodicity should not exceed one year.

This evaluation consists of drawing up a form to assess the availability of equipment and products, compliance with washing, the quality of procedures carried out and compliance with indications.

The form must include at least the following headings:

- Number of beds ;
- Number of water points ;
- Condition of taps ;
- Availability of liquid soap and hydroalcoholic solutions;
- Hand towels and waste bins available,
- Level of infectious risk ;
- Compliance with hand washing or friction ;
- Type of wash complies with instructions ;
- Compliance with the washing or rubbing technique.

V- MAINTENANCE OF HOSPITAL PREMISES

1. INTRODUCTION AND DEFINITIONS

The maintenance of hospital premises helps to reduce the level of environmental contamination and is therefore one of the links in the chain of prevention of nosocomial infections.

Premises maintenance involves cleaning and disinfecting to control the level of microbial contamination in the environment. This includes floors, vertical surfaces (walls and partitions) and horizontal surfaces (worktops, furniture), as well as sanitary facilities.

Biocleaning is defined as a process designed to reduce the biological contamination of surfaces, which is achieved by three actions:

- cleaning ;
- a rinse to remove any dirt and cleaning products used;
- an application of disinfectant.

2. CLASSIFICATION OF PREMISES ACCORDING TO RISK OF INFECTION

A hospital establishment offers a wide variety of premises where hygiene requirements are not identical. Maintenance must take account of this diversity, which depends on the activities carried out, the type of patient admitted and the type of medical procedure performed.

To this end, premises are classified according to the risk of infection into two zones, excluding premises where patients are not admitted.

It is understood that this classification may be modified according to the requirements of each establishment. Desirable requirements for different premises should be discussed internally within the establishment.

Zone 1: **Minimal or medium risk**	Zone 2: **Severe risks**
• Premises receiving patients with - a low or moderate risk of nosocomial infection - • Corridors Lifts Staircases Waiting - rooms • Outpatient consultations - • Functional rehabilitation rooms - Maternity • Psychiatric services - Areas of medical or surgical services not classified as zone 2	Premises for patients with a high risk of nosocomial infection Neonatology Baby-feeding unit Intensive care unit Intensive care unit Emergency department Burns department Transplant department Oncology department Haematology department Paediatrics department Dialysis department Operating theatre Post-operative care room Labour and delivery rooms Minor surgery room Treatment room

	Septic isolation room Analysis laboratory Invasive medical exploration services Interventional medical imaging services

Minimal or medium risk

3. DRESS CODE

Clothing must protect the person in charge of cleaning the premises. It must include at least :

- a tunic and trousers;
- a long-sleeved blouse ;
- a headdress covering the hair ;
- vinyl gloves (household gloves), preferably lined with cotton on the inside;
- waterproof rubber boots.

Gloves and boots must be maintained in the same way as cleaning equipment.

4. CLEANING PRODUCTS

A distinction is made between detergents, disinfectants and detergents and disinfectants. Depending on the case, other products may be used.

4.1.Detergents

A detergent is a product used for cleaning, containing surfactants designed to promote the removal by water of dirt that is not soluble in pure water. Detergents do not destroy micro-organisms by direct action. After using a detergent, surfaces are visually clean but not disinfected.

You can use either 50 milligrams of powder detergent (1/2 cup) diluted in 10 litres of cold water or 30 millilitres of liquid detergent (one measuring cup) diluted in 10 litres of water.

Detergents are commercially available under different names (ISIS®; AIGLE®; BAHDJA®; OMO®; ARIEL®; LE CHAT®...).

4.2.Disinfectants

Disinfection is a temporary operation that eliminates or kills micro-organisms and/or inactivates undesirable viruses carried by contaminated inert media (soil and surfaces).

A disinfectant is a product used for disinfecting inert media, containing at least one active principle with antimicrobial properties. The disinfectant must be used after cleaning. Rinsing is necessary between the application of the detergent and the disinfectant.

The best disinfectant in terms of value for money is bleach, despite its corrosive properties. It comes in two forms:

- 01 litre bottle concentrated to 12° chlorometric; it is used diluted at a dose of 01 litre in 10 litres of water;

- in tubes of A de litre concentrated at 32° chlorometric; it is used diluted at a dose of A de litre in 08 litres of water.

4.3.Detergents and disinfectants

A detergent-disinfectant product has the dual property of detergency and disinfection. In general, these products do not require rinsing.

Two products marketed by laboratories are available on the market: SURFANIOS® and BACTERANIOS D®. They are used diluted at a dose of 20 millilitres in 08 litres of water. These products are packaged in two forms: a 01-litre measuring bottle and a 5-litre can with a metering pump. One dose corresponds to 20 millilitres of product.

4.4.Precautions for use of products

Whatever the product, it is essential to follow the manufacturer's instructions for use, but certain rules must be observed:

- limit the number of products used in the same establishment,
- comply with the technical data sheets ;
- respect the dosages ;
- always use disinfectants on clean surfaces;
- renew diluted solutions every 24 hours;
- always observe a contact time of 20 minutes for disinfectant or detergent and disinfectant solutions;
- respect the peremption dates (from the opening date) ;
- label, date and seal bottles ;
- always use the original packaging;
- always use bleach to check the chlorometric level;
- ensure good stock rotation to avoid obsolescence;
- store away from light, heat and moisture;
- never mix two different products (risk of inactivation or incompatibility, e.g. detergents inactivate bleach).

5. MAINTENANCE EQUIPMENT

The equipment must allow for significant mechanical action. In general, it is necessary to have :

- a scrubber ;
- mops ;
- a push broom ;
- a hand brush ;
- a hand brush ;
- a shovel ;
- 02 or 03 buckets of different colours to distinguish the nature of the solution contained;

- waste collection bags.

The handles of the broom or scrubber should preferably be made of plastic.

The equipment must be cleaned after each use. To do this, prepare a detergent solution, a disinfectant solution and 02 rinsing solutions (tap water). First clean the brushes in the detergent solution, rinse them and then put them in the disinfectant solution for at least 20 minutes. Then rinse them with the second rinsing solution. Repeat the same procedure for the mops.

When you remove the mops from the disinfectant solution and before rinsing them, use one of them to wipe the broom handles. Do not rinse the handles to leave the disinfectant solution in contact with them. Replace the mop in the disinfectant solution and rinse.

Dry brooms and mops in the open air, then store them in a special cupboard.

6. SURFACE MAINTENANCE TECHNIQUES

Because of their simplicity, we have chosen to describe three interview techniques:

6.1. wet sweeping of floors;

6.2. manual floor washing ;

6.3. cleaning and disinfecting surfaces other than floors.

6.4. Wet sweeping of floors

6.4.1. Definition

This operation removes loose dirt from dry, smooth floors.

6.4.2. Objective

Eliminates up to 90% of dust by limiting its suspension in the atmosphere.

6.4.3. Equipment and products

- a scrubber ;
- mops ;
- a bucket ;
- bleach ;
- a waste collection bag.

6.4.4. Technical

- Clearing the ground of large solid or liquid waste;
- Prepare a disinfectant solution (using bleach);
- Dip the first cloth into the disinfectant solution;
- Wring it out;
- Wrap the mop around the cloth;
- Wipe in a single pass and leave to dry;
- Dampen the mop with the disinfectant solution as often as necessary (the mop must be kept damp throughout the operation);
- The mop must rest on the floor at all times to trap waste in front of the

broom;
- Do not lift the scrubber during operation, and do not reverse as this will cause the dirt to be deposited back on the floor;
- Regularly collect the dust and waste collected with the brush and shovel, then place it in the bag;
- Renew the disinfectant solution as often as necessary;
- Change mops between rooms in zone 2 premises;
- Change the mop with the renewal of the solution for zone 1 premises.

Scanning methods :
- Start by sweeping along skirting boards, corners and under furniture;
- Then sweep the free surfaces;
- Push" sweeping for uncluttered areas or corridors;
- Scoop sweeping for cluttered or small areas;
- Always proceed from clean to dirty;
- Finish at the front door.

The "push" method involves sliding the broom in parallel strips in front of you. The "sculling" method involves turning the broom in an S pattern on the floor.

6.4.5. Maintenance schedule

The frequency of maintenance operations varies according to the classification of the premises, the occupancy rate and staff resources. This timetable and the following timetables are given as a guide; each department is free to organise maintenance at its own level.

Zone 1: minimal or medium risk Zone 2: severe risk

Before hand-washing the floors, then every hours on average. 6 hours on average.	Before hand-washing the floors, then every 12 hours on average.

6.5. Manual floor cleaning

6.5.1. Definition

Manual cleaning involves chemical and mechanical action to remove adhering dirt from any waterproof floor.

6.5.2. Objectives

Achieve visual and microbiological cleanliness by reducing the number of micro-organisms present in the soil.

Before any washing, it is necessary to de-clutter the area and wet sweep the floor.

Depending on the type of product used, there are two manual washing methods: the 02-bucket technique and the 03-bucket technique.

6.5.3. The 02-bucket technique

6.5.3.1. Materials and products

- a scrubber ;
- mops ;
- a push broom ;
- 02 buckets of different colours to distinguish the nature of the solution contained ;
- a detergent-disinfectant.

6.5.3.2. Technical

- Prepare the **detergent-disinfectant** solution and the **rinsing** solution (with clean water) in the 02 buckets;
- The buckets must be filled to % to avoid any spillage during the operation;
- Soak the floorcloth in the bucket containing the detergent-disinfectant solution;
- Squeeze lightly over the 2eme bucket containing the rinsing solution;
- Wrap the mop around the cloth;
- Wash the floor using a spatula, with the manipulator always on the dry side;
- For stubborn dirt, use the brush after soaking it in the detergent-disinfectant solution;
- Rinse the mop in the bucket of clean water;
- Squeeze it dry before plunging it back into the detergent-disinfectant solution. Repeat this operation as many times as necessary;
- Leave to dry without rinsing;
- Change the solutions as soon as they become saturated (every 4 rooms on average, i.e. almost 60 to 80 metres^2 ;
- Change mops between rooms in zone 2 premises;
- Change your mop with the renewal of solutions for Zone 1 premises.

6.5.4. The 03-bucket technique

6.5.4.1. Equipment and products

- a scrubber ;
- mops ;
- a push broom ;
- 03 buckets of different colours to distinguish the type of solution contained ;
- a detergent ;
- a disinfectant (bleach).

6.5.4.2. Technical

There are three stages, which must be repeated after each room has been cleaned:

1^{ee} time :

- Prepare the solutions in the 03 buckets: a detergent solution, a disinfectant solution and a rinsing solution (with clean water);
- The buckets must be filled to ¾ to avoid any spillage during the operation;
- Dip the cloth into the bucket containing the detergent solution;
- Squeeze lightly;
- Wrap the mop around the cloth;
- Wash the floor using a spatula, with the manipulator always on the dry side;
- For stubborn dirt, use the brush after soaking it in the detergent solution;
- Rinse the mop in the bucket of clean water;
- Wring it out before dipping it back into the detergent solution. Repeat this operation as many times as necessary.

2ème time:
- Renew the rinsing solution;
- Dip the mop into the bucket;
- Squeeze lightly;
- Wrap the mop around the cloth;
- Always rinse the soil with water;
- Rinse and wring out the mop in the same bucket, repeating this operation as many times as necessary.

For these first two stages, it is necessary to :
- Change the solutions as soon as they become saturated (every 4 rooms on average, i.e. almost 60 a 80 metres^2 ;
- Change mops between rooms in zone 2 premises;
- Change your mop with the renewal of solutions for Zone 1 premises.

3ème time:
- Take the 3eme bucket containing the disinfectant solution;
- Get a new mop;
- Dip the mop into the bucket;
- Squeeze lightly;
- Wrap the mop around the cloth;
- Always wash the soil with water;
- Replace the mop in the bucket as soon as it becomes dry, and repeat the operation as many times as necessary;
- Leave to dry without rinsing.

Once the maintenance of the room is complete, the three steps must be repeated for the next room.

6.5.5. Maintenance schedule

Zone 1: minimal or medium risk	Zone 2: severe risks
Daily.	Daily.

Every other day, apply maintenance Apply   Apply full maintenance (02-bucket technique or complete maintenance (02-bucket technique   03-bucket technique).
or 03-bucket technique).
The other day, apply the first two steps of the 02-bucket technique (detergent removal and ringing without disinfection).

6.6. Cleaning and disinfecting surfaces other than floors

6.6.1. Definition

This operation consists of removing adherent and non-adherent dirt from an impermeable surface other than the floor, by means of chemical and mechanical action.

6.6.2. Objective

Eliminate loose dirt and reduce the number of micro-organisms present on impermeable surfaces. Surfaces may be soiled by splashes of biological fluids or contaminated by hands.

This is particularly important for surfaces that come into contact with hands. It must precede the washing of the floors. The latter must be carried out after the surfaces have been washed.

As with floor washing, there are two different washing methods depending on the type of product used: the 02-bucket technique and the 03-bucket technique.

6.6.3. The 02-bucket technique

6.6.3.1.   Materials and products

* rags (a cloth cut in half will give two rags);
* a hand brush ;
* 02 buckets of different colours to distinguish the nature of the solution contained ;
* a detergent-disinfectant ;
* possibly a stepladder or small ladder.

6.6.3.2.   Technical

* Prepare the detergent-disinfectant solution and the Engage solution (with clean water) in the 02 buckets;
* The buckets must be half full to avoid any spillage during the operation;
* - Dip the cloth into the bucket containing the detergent-disinfectant solution;
* Squeeze lightly over the 2eme bucket containing the rinsing solution;
* Fold it in four;
* Wash surfaces in strips from top to bottom;
* For stubborn stains or irregular surfaces, use the hand brush after dipping it in the bucket containing the detergent-disinfectant solution;
* Rinse the cloth in the bucket of clean water;
* Squeeze it dry before plunging it back into the detergent-disinfectant solution. Repeat this operation as many times as necessary;

- Leave to dry without rinsing;
- Change the solutions as soon as they run out (every 4 rooms on average);
- Change wipes between rooms in zone 2 premises;
- Change wipes with the renewal of solutions for Zone 1 premises.

6.6.4. The 03-bucket technique

6.6.4.1.　　Equipment and products

- rags ;
- a hand brush ;
- 03 buckets of different colours to distinguish the nature of the solution contained ;
- a detergent ;
- a disinfectant (bleach);
- possibly a stepladder or small ladder.

6.6.4.2.　　Technical

There are three stages, which must be repeated after each room has been cleaned:

1^{ee} time:

- Prepare the solutions in the 03 buckets: a detergent solution, a disinfectant solution and a rinsing solution (with clean water);
- The buckets must be half full to avoid any spillage during the operation;
- Dip the cloth into the bucket containing the detergent solution;
- Squeeze lightly;
- Fold it in four;
- Wash surfaces in strips from top to bottom;
- -For stubborn stains or uneven surfaces, use the hand brush after dipping it into the bucket containing the detergent solution;
- Rinse the cloth in the bucket of clean water;
- Wring it out before dipping it back into the detergent solution. Repeat this operation as many times as necessary.

2ème time:

- Renew the rinsing solution;
- Dip the cloth into the bucket;
- Squeeze lightly;
- Fold it in four;
- Always rinse surfaces in strips from top to bottom;
- Rinse and wring out the cloth in the same bucket, repeating this operation as many times as necessary.

For these first two stages, it is necessary to :

- Change the solutions as soon as they run out (every 4 rooms on average);

- Change wipes between rooms in zone 2 premises;
- Change wipes with the renewal of solutions for Zone 1 premises.

3ᵉᵐᵉ time:

- Take the 3ᵉᵐᵉ bucket containing the disinfectant solution;
- Take a new cloth;
- Dip it in the bucket;
- Squeeze lightly;
- Fold it in four;
- Always wash surfaces in strips, from top to bottom;
- Replace the cloth in the bucket as soon as it dries, and repeat the operation as many times as necessary;
- Leave to dry without rinsing.

Once the maintenance of the room is complete, the three steps must be repeated for the next room.

6.6.5. Maintenance schedule

Zone 1: minimal or medium risk	Zone 2: severe risk
Twice a week (02 times a week), Once, apply full maintenance or 03-bucket technique or 03-bucket technique). buckets). The other time, apply the first two steps of the 02-bucket technique (washing and ringing without disinfection).	daily. Apply full maintenance (02-bucket technique or 03-bucket

7. SPECIAL CASES OF PREMISES MAINTENANCE

7.1. Maintenance of sanitary facilities

7.1.1. Definition

Sanitary facilities: washbasins, sinks, showers, baths and toilets are damp places that encourage a high level of microbial proliferation. Their maintenance must take this into account.

7.1.2. Objective

Prevention of infections caused by waterborne germs such as Pseudomonas, Proteus and Serratia.

7.1.3. Equipment and products

- rags ;
- a hand brush ;
- 03 buckets of different colours to distinguish the nature of the solution contained ;
- a detergent ;
- a disinfectant (bleach).

7.1.4. Technical

The operation comprises 03 phases:

1ᵉʳ step: cleaning the outside of the plumbing fixture:
* Prepare the solutions in the 03 buckets: a detergent solution, a disinfectant solution and a rinsing solution (with clean water);
* The buckets must be half full to avoid any spillage during the operation;
* Dip the cloth into the bucket containing the detergent solution;
* Squeeze lightly;
* Fold it in four;
* Wash the outside of the appliance from top to bottom;
* Clean in the following order: wall tiles, paper towel dispenser, underside of appliance, rim, taps, soap dispenser;
* Rinse the cloth;
* Wring it out before dipping it back into the detergent solution. Repeat this operation as many times as necessary.

2ᵉᵐᵉ step: cleaning the inside of the sanitary appliance:
* Pour the rinsing solution back into the sanitary appliance and renew the solution;
* Dip the hand brush into the bucket containing the detergent solution;
* Scrub the inside of the sanitary appliance from clean to dirty;
* Re-dip the brush in the detergent solution as many times as necessary;
* Pour the rinsing solution back into the plumbing fixture;
* Renew the rinsing solution;
* Soak the cloth in the bucket of clean water;
* Squeeze lightly;
* Fold it in four;
* Rinse all surfaces (outside then inside), always from top to bottom and in the same order;
* Rinse and wring out the cloth in the same bucket, repeating this operation as many times as necessary.

It is necessary for these 02 times to :
* Change the solutions as soon as they run out;
* Change the cloth between each sanitary appliance;
* Clean and disinfect the hand brush between each sanitary appliance.

3ᵉᵐᵉ time: disinfection of the sanitary equipment :
* Take the 3ᵉᵐᵉ bucket containing the disinfectant solution;
* Take a new cloth;
* Dip it in the bucket;
* Squeeze lightly;
* Fold it in four;
* Wash interior and exterior surfaces, always from top to bottom and in the

same order;

- Replace the cloth in the bucket as soon as it dries, and repeat the operation as many times as necessary;
- Leave to dry without rinsing;
- Pour the contents of a glass of 12°C chlorine bleach (200 millilitres) inside the siphon and any overflow, and leave in contact for at least 10 minutes.

7.1.5. Maintenance schedule

Washrooms must be cleaned daily, whatever the classification of the premises. This should be followed by a floor wash.

7.2.Operating theatre maintenance

7.2.1. Definition

Operating theatres are places where procedures with a very high risk of infection are carried out, requiring rigorous aseptic conditions.

The maintenance of these premises should establish a coherent relationship between the environment and the actions carried out there.

7.2.2. Objective

To achieve ultra-clean operating theatres and annexes.

7.2.3. Equipment and products

- rags ;
- mops ;
- a scrubber ;
- 02 or 03 buckets in different colours depending on the technique used;
- a detergent-disinfectant or, failing that, a detergent and a disinfectant (bleach);
- possibly a stepladder or small ladder.

7.2.4. Technical

The techniques described above should be used for cleaning and disinfecting surfaces. For surfaces other than floors, another technique will be used: wet wiping.

Wet wiping is an operation designed to remove loose dirt. The technique is as follows:

- Prepare a detergent-disinfectant solution or, failing that, a disinfectant solution (using bleach);
- Dip the cloth into the solution;
- Wring it out;
- Fold in quarters and wipe dry in a single pass;
- Dampen the cloth with the solution as many times as necessary;
- Leave to dry;
- Proceed from clean to dirty and from top to bottom.

The use of bleach is not recommended because of its corrosive action on metallic materials.

7.2.5. Maintenance schedule

7.2.5.1.   Before the operation

Start by wiping the operating table and horizontal surfaces (top of operating table, arm rest, instrument table, gueridon, stool top, etc.) with a damp cloth.

Then wipe the anaesthetic equipment (anaesthetic table, scope, respirator, defibrillator, syringe pump, etc.) with a damp cloth.

Follow this up with a damp sweep of the floor.

7.2.5.2.   Between interventions

The work is entrusted to one or two people at most.

Disposing of dirty linen, suction jars, instruments and waste (emptying rubbish bins, cleaning and disinfecting them, disposing of rubbish bags and replacing them).

Change the suction jars.

Wet-wipe the horizontal surfaces (table and armrests, instrument table, operating theatre handle, etc.).

Then wash the floor.

Wait until the floor is dry before entering the room.

In an emergency, replace floor washing with wet sweeping.

7.2.5.3.   At the end of the day

Carry out the same procedures as between interventions, completed by the following steps:

• Washing of all surfaces other than floors and ceilings (fixed horizontal surfaces and walls);

• Washing of annexes (preparation rooms for the surgeon and surgeon, sterile arsenals, recovery room if coiitigucv...).

7.2.5.4.   Once a week or after a septic procedure

Carry out the same procedures as at the end of the day, completed by the following steps:

• Wet wiping of air vents and ultraviolet lamp reflectors ;

• Wet wiping ceilings ;

• Airborne disinfection.

7.3. Other specific maintenance requirements for certain premises

In traffic areas (corridors, staircases, entrance halls, etc.) where traffic can be very heavy, floors should be cleaned several times a day. Wet sweeping of floors is preferred. To allow people to pass through, always clean in half. Wet wipe surfaces frequently in contact with hands (door handles, handrails, etc.).

For patient rooms, the cleaning schedule must take into account nursing care, medical interventions and room contamination. Always start cleaning with the least contaminated rooms. Potted flowers are forbidden in all departments and cut flowers in zone 2 rooms. Flower water should be changed daily and lightly bleached (01 teaspoon of 12° chlorometric bleach).

8. ASSESSMENT OF PREMISES MAINTENANCE

8.1. Audit assessment

An audit may be organised periodically by the medical supervisor or the hygiene department of the establishment. The periodicity should not exceed one quarter.

This evaluation consists of drawing up a form containing an assessment of all or some of the stages in the maintenance of the premises.

The form must include at least the following headings:

- Period of the interview ;
- Wearing of protective clothing by the cleaner ;
- Availability of the necessary equipment;
- Respect the dilution dose of products ;
- Compliance with maintenance techniques ;
- Respect the contact time of the disinfectant solution ;
- Disinfection of equipment after use.

8.2. Microbiological evaluation

In order to assess the effectiveness of biocleaning, regular microbiological sampling of surfaces may be carried out 01 time per quarter only in operating theatres or sterile isolation rooms in haemato-oncology. These samples must be taken by competent persons, and cooperation between the hygiene department and the establishment's microbiology laboratory is necessary for this purpose.

VI- TREATMENT OF MEDIC AUX DEVICES

1. INTRODUCTION AND DEFINITIONS

The general term "medical devices" covers a wide range of equipment used for a variety of purposes: prevention, screening, diagnosis and treatment.

Once contaminated with germs from the patient and/or the environment, this medical and surgical equipment must undergo various treatments before being put back into circulation, each stage having its own specificity. This treatment will be carried out after assessing the level of infectious risk.

Disinfecting or sterilising clean equipment eliminates the pathogenic organisms present and prevents them from being transmitted by this equipment to other patients, members of staff or the environment.

2. ASSESSMENT OF THE RISK OF INFECTION AND THE LEVEL OF TREATMENT REQUIRED DEPENDING ON THE INTENDED USE OF THE EQUIPMENT

Three levels of infectious risk are defined according to the nature of the tissue with which the medical device comes into contact during use. These levels correspond to defined levels of treatment, enabling the required level of microbiological quality to be achieved.

Destination of the material	Equipment classification	Level of infectious risk	Treatment level
Introduction into the vascular system or into a cavity or sterile tissue by any route. *Examples: surgical instruments, implants, arthroscopes, small dressing instruments*	Review	High risk	Sterilisation or single use or, failing that, high-level disinfection (if sterilisation impossible or single use non-existent)
In contact with mucous membranes or superficially lesioned skin. *Examples: gastroscopes, colonoscopes*	Semi-critical	Median risk	Intermediate-level disinfection
In contact with intact skin d^u patient or without contact with No c.^ Low risk to the patient *Examples: blood pressure monitors, beds*			Low-level disinfection

3. GENERAL CIRCUIT FOR PROCESSING MEDICAL DEVICES

The circuit comprises 4 equally important stages:

* Pre-disinfection ;
* Cleaning;

- Sterilisation or disinfection;
- Storage.

3.1.Predesinfection

3.1.1. Objectives

Remove dirt (particularly organic matter: pus, blood, secretions, etc.), reduce micro-organisms and make cleaning easier. This step avoids the fixation of organic matter by drying, contamination of personnel and contamination of the environment.

3.1.2. Equipment and products

- Containers with sufficient volume for the quantity of devices to be immersed;
- Detergent-disinfectant product or, failing that, a detergent only (these products and their instructions for use are described in detail in the "Cleaning hospital premises" chapter);
- Water from the network.

3.1.3. Technical

- Fill the trays with the detergent-disinfectant solution or, failing that, with a detergent-only solution;
- Immediately after use, immerse the treatment devices at the point of use;
- Wipe off medical devices that cannot be soaked;
- For medical devices with cavities, it is imperative to irrigate the channels in order to remove dirt immediately.

3.2.Cleaning

3.2.1. Objectives

Eliminate dirt and reduce the number of micro-organisms present on the equipment. This stage combines the physico-chemical action of the product (detergent), the thermal action and the mechanical action of brushing (and/or swabbing) and rinsing.

3.2.2. Equipment and products

- Containers with sufficient volume for the quantity of devices to be immersed;
- Detergent-disinfectant product or detergent only;
- Water from the network ;
- Wipes, brushes, toothbrushes, swabs ;
- Dry, lint-free, clean cloth, disinfects between 2 uses.

3.2.3. Technical

- Fill the trays with the detergent-disinfectant solution or, failing that, with a detergent-only solution;
- Immerse the equipment;

- Brushing and swabbing the canals;
- Rinse thoroughly with mains water;

Pre-disinfection followed by cleaning is sufficient for low-risk disinfection. Otherwise, this initial treatment should be completed by sterilisation or by high-level or intermediate-level disinfection.

Drying is carried out at the end of this phase, unless the devices are intended for high-level or intermediate-level disinfection. The objectives of drying are to limit microbial proliferation during storage and to limit the risk of rust. It is carried out using a dry cloth or compressed air.

3.3.Sterilisation

3.3.1. Objectives

Eliminate all living micro-organisms and maintain sterility through packaging.

3.3.2. Equipment and products

- Autoclave: steam steriliser.

Dry heat sterilisation processes *(such as poupinel)* should no longer be used due to poor internal distribution of the sterilising agent and their ineffectiveness on non-conventional transmissible agents *(prions)*.

3.3.3. Technical

3.3.3.1.   Packaging

It must be chosen according to the medical device to be sterilised and must guarantee sterility after passing through the steriliser and throughout the storage period. It may take the form of :
- Single or double bags;
- Crepe paper always in double thickness;
- Unwoven paper ;
- Containers (rigid, reusable packaging).

3.3.3.2.   Stages of sterilisation

Bowie-Dick test

This is the first test to be carried out before the first sterilisation of the day. This test verifies the ability of the steam to penetrate a standard load, and the elimination of air (i.e. indirectly the absence of leakage). For this purpose, either packs made on site or ready-to-use Bowie-Dick test packs are used. Once the pack has been made up, it is placed on its own in the tank. A textile cycle at 134°C / 3.5 minutes is then started. This cycle is pre-programmed on recent machines.

Interpretation of the test: After observing the test in direct light, the colour change of the ink (= colour change over the entire surface) after exposure to 134°C / 3.5 minutes should be homogeneous.

If the cycle does not conform, a lighter spot appears in the centre of the sheet. In this case, the steam has not penetrated to the heart of the pack; the temperature is higher.

the sterile state is not guaranteed. The appliance cannot therefore be used and the intervention of a technician is necessary.

Load preparation

Build up a homogeneous load by placing the material in baskets with a layout that facilitates steam penetration. Take care a :

- place the containers at the bottom ;
- Place the individual sachets vertically in the baskets and do not pack them;
- the load must occupy a maximum of 70% of the total volume of the tank.

Place the physico-chemical indicators in the load to be sterilised. These indicators respond to the three parameters of time, temperature and presence of water vapour. Class 6 indicators (standard ISO 11 140-1), also known as cycle verification indicators or emulation indicators, are used. They are placed in each container or bag, or distributed in geometrically shaped test packs (minimum 5 per load). Whatever the choice, they must always be placed inside the packaging.

Loading

Choose the appropriate cycle according to the material to be sterilised, as steam injections and tray duration vary from one cycle to another: instrument cycle (134°C/18min), linen cycle (134°C / 18 min or less depending on validation), rubber cycle (125°C / 20 min).

Load into the autoclave and start the sterilisation cycle. The cycle parameters are set automatically.

Download

Remove the trolley, allow the load to cool, collect the indicators and carry out the post-sterilisation checks.

3.3.3.3. Sterilisation control and evaluation

Contrôles before sterilisation

Check the operation of the appliance and the water supply. Carry out a Bowie-Dick test every morning.

Contrôles during sterilisation

Check pressure gauges, thermometers, cycle phases and correct cycle operation (alarms).

Contrôles after sterilisation

Check that items have passed through the steriliser by turning the passage indicators. Passage indicators are used to identify items that have passed through the autoclave but are not a sterility check.

3.4.Disinfection

3.4.1. Objectives

Operation with a momentary result, enabling micro-organisms to be eliminated or killed and/or undesirable viruses carried on contaminated inert media to be inactivated, depending on the objectives set (e.g. 5 log reduction in the bacterial population). The result of this operation is limited to the micro-organisms present at the time of the operation.

Disinfection is ephemeral and should never replace sterilisation when the critical material is heat-resistant.

3.4.2. Equipment and products

* Protective clothing: gloves, goggles, mask, overblouse or protective apron;
* 1 Immersion tank ;
* 1 rinsing tank ;
* 20 millilitre syringes ;
* Disinfectant solution ;
* Air medical filter ;
* Dry, lint-free, clean or sterile cloth as appropriate;
* Sterile field ;
* Sterile water, bacteriologically controlled water or mains water.

The disinfectants available are :

* Glutaraldehyde a 2%, marketed under different trade names by the pharmacie centrale des hopitaux and marketed by ANIOS/NOSOCLEAN laboratories under the name STERANIOS®.
* Bleach a 12°chlorimetric, should only be used exceptionally and in an emergency due to its highly corrosive effect on medical devices.

3.4.3. Technical

* Wear protective clothing ;
* Fill the tray with the disinfectant solution;
* Fill the second tank with the rinsing solution;
* Immerse the equipment in the disinfectant solution. The immersion time depends on the spectrum of activity required (15 minutes for bactericidal and virucidal action, 60 minutes for sporicidal action);
* Irrigate the canals with the disinfectant solution using the syringe;
* Remove the equipment from the disinfectant solution and place it in the rinsing solution;
* Rinse thoroughly, purging the canals with the syringe.

Use for rinsing:

* Network water for medical devices intended for digestive endoscopy;
* Bacteriologically controlled water for medical devices intended a for

bronchial endoscopy procedures;

• Sterile water for medical devices intended for sterile cavities.

Rinsing of disinfected medical devices is followed by drying and storage.

Drying is carried out using filtered medical air and/or a dry cloth, sterile if rinsing with sterile or bacteriologically controlled water, or clean if rinsing with mains water.

Wrap the medical device in a sterile drape and indicate the date and time of disinfection.

Any equipment disinfected after a high-level or intermediate-level procedure, and stored for >12 hours, must undergo a new disinfection procedure before being reused.

3.5.Storage

3.5.1. Objectives

Keep disinfected equipment intact and prevent recontamination.

3.5.2. Technical

Store sterilised or disinfected equipment in a **clean, closed and regularly disinfected** cupboard.

VII- HOSPITAL LINEN CIRCUIT

1. INTRODUCTION AND DEFINITIONS

Hospital linen is a necessary element in both technical care and nursing, and is a permanent feature of hospital life. It is easily and very quickly contaminated when it comes into contact with patients, and can be contaminated when it is disposed of.

After use, linen is always contaminated either by saprophytic and commensal germs, or by pathogenic germs, reflecting the hospital service's ecosystem.

Linen care comprises 2 separate circuits, one dirty and the other clean. The dirty circuit begins with the collection of soiled linen and ends with its arrival at the laundry. The clean circuit starts at the laundry and continues until it is used by the patient or nursing staff.

2. NATURE OF HOSPITAL LINEN

The nature of hospital linen has changed considerably in recent years, in response to economic constraints, infectious risk prevention and patient comfort. Cotton is now giving way to polyester/cotton blends or pure polyester, because they are easy to clean and act as a barrier to micro-organisms.

The most common dosages are :

- 65% polyester - 35% cotton : Vetements hospitaliers ;
- 50% polyester - 50% cotton : Bed linen, surgical drapes, gowns ;
- 35% polyester - 65% cotton : Technical clothing, kitchen clothing.

3. DIRTY LINEN CIRCUIT

This tour includes the following stages:

- pick-up ;
- sorting ;
- intermediate storage ;
- transport to the laundry.

3.1.Collection

Soiled linen is collected after each bed change and during the patient's grooming and body care.

Collected linen is taken out into the corridor (outside patients' rooms or treatment rooms). Care should be taken to remove all items that should not be sent to the laundry, such as diapers and/or protective clothing, dental or hearing aids, pens and other vulnerable items. These items can damage the machines and pose a risk to laundry staff.

Soiled linen must be handled using single-use non-sterile vinyl gloves.

3.2.Sorting

Once taken to the corridor, the laundry is sorted into 4 categories:

• White linen (bed sheet, mattress cover, bedspread, pillowcase, towel, flannel, tea towel, etc.);

• Fragile linen (blankets, etc.) ;

• Coloured linen (operating theatre linen and risk services) ;

• Shaped linen (pyjama jacket, pyjama trousers, nightdress, operating gown, surgeon's gown, etc.).

Each category is placed in a plastic bag (bin bag). The bags must be of different colours so that they can be identified in the laundry before being put in the machine. Once the bags have been filled to capacity, they are sealed with a string.

3.3.Intermediate storage

Once the bags have been filled, they are transported on a trolley either to a cupboard reserved for this purpose or to a specific room. They should not be stored for more than 48 hours.

Laundry must never be stored on the floor.

Once unloaded, the trolley must be disinfected. The cupboard or room is disinfected at least once a week.

3.4.Transport to the laundry

The linen is taken to the laundry either by trolley if it is close to the department concerned, or by vehicle if it is located outside the establishment.

The trolley or vehicle must be absolutely disinfected after unloading, especially if it is used to transport clean linen from the laundry to the user departments.

4. LINEN TREATMENT

The dirty linen arrives in the "dirty" area of the laundry (a room reserved for the reception and temporary storage of dirty linen). The linen then undergoes several treatments:

• Insect repellent may be required;

• Pre-disinfection;

• Machine wash ;

• A rinse ;

• Drying;

• Ironing if required;

• A fold.

Desinsectisation is used when linen is infested by ectoparasites or insects (lice, fleas, bedbugs, etc.).

Pre-disinfection is carried out using a disinfectant solution. A specific disinfectant for linen such as STERILINGE®, marketed by

ANIOS/NOSOCLEAN laboratories, should be used for this purpose. Alternatively, bleach can be used in an appropriate concentration (as described in the section on "Cleaning hospital premises").

Once the linen has been processed, it is put into plastic bags (bin bags) to be used as packaging until it can be reused.

5. CLEAN LINEN CIRCUIT

Bags of clean linen are temporarily stored in the "clean" area of the laundry (clean linen room) until they are delivered to the user departments.

This clean linen is always handled by disinfected hands (practice regular hygienic hand washing).

Linen is transported in trolleys or a disinfected vehicle to the wards, or stored in a cupboard or wardrobe reserved for this purpose. Linen must not be unpacked until it has been used by the patient or nursing staff.

The clean and dirty linen circuits must never meet.

VIII- MANAGEMENT OF HEALTHCARE WASTE

1. INTRODUCTION AND DEFINITIONS

Healthcare waste is defined as waste from diagnostic, monitoring and preventive, curative or palliative treatment activities in the field of human and veterinary medicine. There are 2 types of waste: household waste and infectious risk waste. Responsibility for managing infectious risk waste lies with the establishment that produces it (the healthcare organisation) until it is disposed of.

Infectious risk healthcare waste (IRHW) is waste soiled with blood or biological material (faeces, urine, vomit, pus, etc.), dressings, single-use equipment or equipment used for patients in isolation, laboratory equipment (tubes, culture media, etc.), sharp objects (syringe needles, scalpel blades, etc.), anatomical parts (organs, placentas, etc.).

Even though it represents only a small proportion of all waste in hospitals, HIW needs to be managed in a very specific way because of the risks it can pose to the health of patients, carers and the environment. These risks may be

trauma (injury by sharp objects) or nosocomial infections (multi-resistant germ infections, viral hepatitis B or C, HIV).

In this presentation, we will distinguish between two types of HIW: sharps and soft infectious risk waste, which does not present a traumatic risk.

2. WASTE DISPOSAL CIRCUIT, ITS OBJECTIVES AND THE EQUIPMENT NEEDED TO CARRY IT OUT

There are four stages in the management of waste, from its production by hospital staff to its disposal:

- Collection ;
- Storage ;
- Transport ;
- Treatment.

2.1. Collection

2.1.1. Objective

Sorting waste at the production stage so that it can be disposed of while protecting the people involved in the process.

2.1.2. Equipment required

- Rigid, leak-proof yellow plastic containers bearing a specific pictogram. The lid must be tamper-proof when closed;

- 2 different coloured bin liners (yellow and black);
- Strings ;
- If necessary, bin holders or plastic bins.

If yellow or black refuse bags are not available, other colours can be chosen, provided that information is given about the specific characteristics of each colour. Red could be chosen for example for DASRI and green for household waste.

2.1.3. Technical

The waste is collected at the place where it is produced after a care activity (treatment room, operating theatre, patient rooms, etc.). The waste producer must sort the waste according to its type:

- Sharps waste must be disposed of after use and without any unnecessary handling in the sealed containers.
- Other infectious risk waste must be disposed of in yellow bin bags.
- Non-infectious household waste must be disposed of in black bin bags. Glass waste is treated as household waste.

This initial sorting of waste is vital for the rest of the healthcare waste disposal chain.

Bags that are being filled must not be left on the floor in the departments. They should be placed either on racks or in plastic bins. Disinfect this support with bleach at least once a week using the wet wiping technique.

2.2.Storage

2.2.1. Objective

Temporary storage of waste previously packaged and sorted for one or more care units for the same service, with a view to transport.

2.2.2. Equipment required

Large-volume plastic bins with lids and wheels, container type, the number of which will depend on the volume of waste produced by the service.

2.2.3. Technical

- Once the containers are 3/4 full, they are sealed with tamper-proof lids, and once the yellow and black bin liners are 2/3 full, they are sealed with a string that must be resistant to subsequent handling.
- Watertight containers and yellow bags will be separated from black bags and placed in containers bearing a pictogram indicating the infectious risk of their contents.
- Black bags can be stored away from patients and nursing staff.

Disinfect containers with bleach at least once a month.

2.3. Transport

2.3.1. Equipment required

A specific collection vehicle (van type).

2.3.2. Technical

• The transport and management of the black bags are the responsibility of the company responsible for waste collection by the local authority.

• The hospital's environmental department is responsible for disposing of the hazardous waste contained in the sealed containers and yellow bags. This type of waste is collected and transported on a daily basis. A collection schedule should be drawn up between the department producing the waste and the environment department. DASRI must be stored outside the department just before the collection vehicle arrives, to prevent any infectious risk that could be caused by close contact with this type of waste. It is imperative for those concerned to respect the collection schedule.

2.4. Disposal of hazardous waste

2.4.1. Objective

The transformation of hazardous waste into non-hazardous waste in order to limit its impact on human health and the environment.

2.4.2. Equipment required

- Pyrolytic incinerator.

This incinerator should preferably be located outside the hospital and meet current anti-pollution standards. It may be shared by several hospitals.

2.4.3. Technical

DASRI is sent by the environment department to the incinerator. Incineration at 1000°C transforms infectious risk waste into non-hazardous waste and considerably reduces its volume.

It should be remembered that incineration only concerns DASRI, so the initial sorting of waste as soon as it is produced is essential.

It is therefore imperative that the watertight containers and yellow bags should only contain DASRI.

2.4.4. Other techniques for disposing of hazardous waste

In the absence of a pyrolytic incinerator, three other techniques can be used: trivialisation, simple incineration and landfill.

2.4.4.1.   Commonplace

Banalisation is a process for transforming medical waste into waste similar to household refuse. This process uses equipment that crushes and then disinfects the medical waste. The product obtained in this way can be transported by the company responsible for waste collection via the local authority services responsible for the area.

2.4.4.2.   Simple incineration

DASRI is placed in a metal drum with a capacity of at least 500 litres. Incineration is carried out by spraying with fuel oil or kerosene. The opening of the drum must be protected by a metal grille to contain any splashes. This low-temperature incineration (£ 200°C) eliminates almost 99% of micro-organisms.

2.4.4.3.   Landfill

DASRI can be buried on land belonging to the hospital establishment or on land granted by the municipal services for this purpose. The soil must be impermeable, preferably clay. The pit must be large enough to contain the volume of waste produced in one month's activity.

The pit must be surrounded by a fence high enough to prevent access by anyone outside the service.

Once the pit has been filled to the top, it should be covered with a thick layer of clay to act as a barrier against bad weather.

3. EVALUATION OF THE DASRI DISPOSAL CIRCUIT

In order to be able to estimate the volume of HIW produced by the CHU's departments and to assess compliance with sorting during the initial collection from these departments, a labelling system for watertight containers and yellow bags should be put in place. This labelling will include the name of the department, the name of the unit and the date of disposal.

This labelling will make it possible to check that the waste producer has sorted the waste at the time of collection. Checks should be carried out before the waste is disposed of.

The volume of hazardous waste should not exceed 1/5 of the total volume of healthcare waste. Any excess will indicate non-compliance with the initial sorting.

IX- PREVENTION OF SURGICAL SITE INFECTIONS

1. INTRODUCTION

Surgical site infections are a frequent complication of surgical procedures. At the Blida University Hospital Centre, they accounted for almost half of all nosocomial infections in 2003 and 2004, making it the leading hospital in terms of nosocomial infections. In developed countries, SSIs account for 10% of all hospital-acquired infections. They can have serious consequences, even threatening the patient's vital prognosis.

The prevention of these frequent and serious infections depends on the quality of the patient's pre-operative skin preparation, as any cutaneous incision may constitute a source of infection There are two fundamental aspects to this preparation: body hygiene and skin and mucous membrane disinfection of the surgical site. The practice of depilating the operating area is highly debatable.

2. BODY HYGIENE

2.1.Brushing the teeth

Tooth brushing is essential for all operations. In cardiac and oral surgery, antiseptic mouthwashes are recommended before and after the operation.

2.2.Pre-operative toilet

The shower (or toilet for dependent patients) reduces the microbial flora and facilitates the subsequent action of the antiseptic used to disinfect the operating field. At least one pre-operative shower is recommended. The patient is helped according to his or her autonomy. For dependent patients, the use of a shower trolley is preferred to washing in bed.

A foaming polyvidone-iodine-based antiseptic solution such as Betadine® Foaming or its equivalent should be used for this purpose. It is recommended that the antiseptic used should always be from the same family, from the first shower to the last application of antiseptic in the operating theatre.

Showering should be carried out no more than 3 hours before the operation or, failing that, the day before to minimise recontamination of the skin.

Before showering, it is necessary to remove jewellery, wedding rings, piercings, varnish, make-up, etc.

Always wash from the cleanest to the most contaminated area. Start with the face, neck, chest, back, limbs, feet, armpits and then the genito-anal area.

After the shower, the patient's clothing should be changed and the bed made up with clean linen. It is recommended that the patient be dressed in a single-use cap, or failing that, in a clean cloth cap.

3. DEPILATION

The aim of depilation is to cut the hair at the base when it is troublesome for the operation or for the dressing. It must be carried out without weighing down the skin. Mechanical shaving is a risky method and should be avoided.

Depilation is not essential; on the contrary, not depilating the surgical area is the simplest and safest solution, as long as it does not affect the per- and post-operative imperatives.

If depilation is deemed unavoidable, the technique chosen must be non-aggressive. Either mowing (with clippers) or chemical depilation (with depilatory cream) will be used.

Hair removal should be carried out as close as possible to the operation. It is not advisable to have the hair removed in the operating theatre.

4. SKIN AND MUCOUS MEMBRANE DISINFECTION OF THE OPERATING SITE

The aim of disinfecting the operating site is to reduce the number of micro-organisms present on the surgeon's skin and/or mucosa, to avoid contamination of the incision by micro-organisms present at the site and throughout the operation, in order to prevent infection of the operating site.

Cutaneous preparation of the operating field must be thorough. It comprises 04 stages: detersion, rinsing, drying and dermal antisepsis.

4.1.Detersion

The aim of preoperative detersion is to reduce bacterial contamination and cutaneous scales and debris on the skin in the incision area, before applying the antiseptic. It should be carried out after showering or washing in bed, preferably within the hour before surgery, to limit the risk of recolonisation of the surgical site.

A foaming antiseptic solution such as Betadine® foam or its equivalent is used for detersion.

Always start detersion at the incision line. In the case of multiple operating areas, start with the highest and/or cleanest area. Apply circularly using a sterile compress soaked in sterile water and the foaming antiseptic solution.

For cranial surgery without shearing, apply a shampoo containing the antiseptic solution.

4.2.Rinsing

Rinse thoroughly with sterile water and sterile compresses.

4.3.Drying

Drying is always done by swabbing with sterile compresses.

4.4.Dermal antisepsis

Antisepsis must be carried out immediately after drying. Use an antiseptic from the same range as the product used for showering and cleansing, such as Betadine® d 10%.

For patients being prepared in the operating theatre, dermal antisepsis consists of applying 2 successive swabs. It is important to respect the drying time between the 2 swabs.

For patients prepared on the ward, the first application of antiseptic is carried out in the unit, with 2 further applications in the operating theatre.

Whatever the case, the dressing must extend well beyond the incision line and take into account the possible placement of drains. In the operating theatre, it must be carried out by a member of the team in surgical clothing, using cups, forceps, compresses and sterile gloves.

Brushing is applied to healthy skin from the operating area towards the periphery. On an infected wound or surgical site with significant microbial proliferation (perianal area for example), it should be applied from the periphery towards the surgical site.

The skin incision is only made when the second antiseptic dressing has dried.

5. DRAPING THE PATIENT

Draping the operating area in a sterile drape is not recommended, as it accelerates microbial recolonisation. However, if draping is necessary, non-woven textiles should be used. The use of 100% cotton textiles is strictly prohibited.

X-PREVENTION OF URINARY TRACT INFECTIONS

1. INTRODUCTION

Urinary tract infections account for almost 40% of hospital-acquired infections in developed countries, making them the leading cause. At Blida University Hospital Centre, they also accounted for almost 4 out of 10 nosocomial infections in the prevalence surveys carried out between 2001 and 2004, and ranked second after surgical site infections.

The main risk factor is urinary catheterisation, which is often carried out in wards with a high risk of nosocomial infection.

The prevention of these frequent infections depends on compliance with the indications for urinary catheterisation and the insertion technique, as well as on the quality of maintenance and management of the system.

2. INDICATIONS AND DURATION OF THE SURVEY

The indications and duration of indwelling bladder catheterisation must be kept to a minimum and always on medical prescription. The indication must be reconsidered every day. The most valid indications are :

- urinary obstruction ;
- urogenital tract surgery ;
- a medical cause requiring diuresis monitoring;
- prevention of maceration and sacral eschar infection in bedridden patients.

The catheter should be removed as soon as it is no longer required. An alternative to permanent bladder catheterisation is always preferable, i.e. penis covers, absorbent nappies, etc.

3. PREVENTION DURING THE SURVEY

Inserting a catheter through the urinary tract to the bladder, following the path of the ureter, is an invasive procedure with a potential risk of infection. The insertion of a urinary catheter must follow 16 compulsory steps.

1. The equipment is placed on a previously cleaned and disinfected surface with clean hands (simple hand washing). Use a special bin liner.

2. Before insertion, perform a genital cleansing. The operator must use single-use non-sterile gloves. Start by soaping the perineal area using a foaming antiseptic solution based on polyvidone-iodine such as Betadine® foaming solution or its equivalent. If this is not available, use a mild liquid soap. It is recommended that the antiseptic used is always from the same family from the first to the last application of antiseptic. After soaping, rinse thoroughly with

clean water and dry.

3. Then wash your hands hygienically or, better still, disinfect them by friction with a hydro-alcoholic solution on hands that are not macroscopically soiled.

4. Place the catheter, collection bag, antiseptic-soaked swabs (10% Betadine® type polyvidone-iodine), sterile lubricant-soaked swabs (Vaseline and paraffin oil are not recommended because of the risk of damaging the catheter), sterile water, sterile 10-millilitre syringe and sterile split drape (preferably single-use) on the sterile drape on the table.

5. Apply antisepsis to the meat (with forceps), always working from top to bottom.

6. Wear single-use sterile gloves.

7. Lubricate the probe and adapt it to the collection bag. From this point on, the bag will never be maladjusted for the duration of the catheterisation.

8. Fill the syringe with sterile water and check the balloon.

9. Place the split drape over the patient.

10. Probe the patient.

11. Inflate the balloon with the syringe of sterile water (volume indicated on the probe).

12. Remove the split field, equipment and gloves.

13. Secure the catheter with a plaster, on the abdomen in men and on the thigh in women.

14. Hang the collection bag sloping down in relation to the bladder.

15. Hygienic hand washing or disinfection by friction with a hydro-alcoholic solution.

16. Note the date of application on the treatment form.

4. PREVENTION LINKED TO MAINTENANCE OF THE CLOSED SYSTEM

Care adapted to patients with an indwelling bladder catheter reduces the risk of urinary tract infection. The overall quality of this care is based on the patient's body hygiene, the operator's hand hygiene and absolute respect for closed drainage.

4.1. Hand hygiene

All care given to patients undergoing catheterisation must be preceded and followed by hygienic hand washing or, better still, disinfection by friction with a hydro-alcoholic solution on hands that are not macroscopically soiled.

4.2. Strict compliance with enclosed drainage

The catheter and collection bag remain attached throughout the catheterisation process. They are removed together (clamped collection bag). Urine samples are taken aseptically from the ring provided for this purpose.

4.3.Maintaining urine flow

The urine must flow freely into the collection bag. This is positioned sloping down in relation to the level of the bladder. Hydration of the patient is essential in order to obtain a urine output of at least 1.5 litres per day (unless medically contraindicated).

4.4.Local care

Genital cleansing should be carried out at least once a day, and after each bowel movement. A mild liquid soap is used, followed by a thorough rinse with water. A catheterised patient may take a shower. Make sure the catheter is correctly attached beforehand.

4.5.Emptying the collection bag

The collection bag is emptied regularly: do not exceed 2/3. The drainage tap is decontaminated before opening, using a compress soaked in antiseptic. While the urine is flowing, the tap is not in contact with the collection jar. The jar is cleaned and disinfected once a day.

4.6.Vesical irrigation

Systematic bladder washing is of no use in preventing catheter-associated urinary tract infections. In fact, the practice is harmful. It can only be tolerated in cases of absolute necessity, and only if the bladder catheter is a dual-current catheter.

It should be noted that the local application of an antiseptic is an ineffective and sometimes damaging measure.

4.7.General surveillance

Urinary tract infection is asymptomatic from the outset. Temperature monitoring, at least once a day, is therefore an important part of general monitoring. The volume and appearance of the urine should be noted daily.

4.8.Incidents

If the probe is blocked, change it. Never try to unblock it.

If there is a leak in the collection bag, change the bag without changing the catheter, taking all the necessary aseptic precautions.

XI- INFECTION PREVENTION PULMONARY

1. INTRODUCTION

Lung infections account for almost 20% of hospital-acquired infections in developed countries. At Blida University Hospital, they also accounted for almost 2 out of 10 nosocomial infections in the prevalence surveys carried out between 2001 and 2004, ranking third after surgical site infections and urinary tract infections.

However, their frequency is much higher in certain high-risk departments where invasive respiratory procedures are performed. Monitoring over 6 months in the general intensive care unit at Beni-Messous University Hospital (Algiers) revealed a cumulative incidence of almost 50%, placing this type of infection well ahead of urinary tract infections and bacteremia/septicemia. The risk factors for these infections are related either to the patient himself, or to the equipment, or to the environment.

2. RISK FACTORS

2.1.2-1- Patient-related factors

- Student age ;
- Presence of associated diseases (diabetes, IITA...) ;
- Presence of primary or acquired immunodepression (through treatment, for example);
- The seriousness of his condition;
- Use of sedatives (which cause a reduction or loss of reflexes in the upper airways and encourage the inhalation of rhino-pharyngeal secretions);
- Presence of a gastric or enteral feeding tube;
- The decubitus position ;
- Modification of oropharyngeal flora.

2.2. Equipment-related factors

- Placement of an intubation or tracheostomy tube ;
- Endotracheal suction ;
- Bronchial endoscopy ;
- Respiratory assistance.

2.3. Environmental factors

Most often transmitted by hand. All environmental factors can be responsible: floors and surfaces, laundry, air, water, etc.

3. PREVENTIVE MEASURES

In addition to basic hygiene measures, specific hygiene measures must be observed.

3.1.Basic measures

The basic measures are :

- washing hands after any contact with contaminated secretions or materials, particularly when performing oropharyngeal and bronchial aspirations;
- Wearing a mask during treatment involving the splashing or spraying of biological fluids;
- the use of sterile equipment or equipment that has undergone an appropriate disinfection procedure;
- the use of sterile water. The bottle opened at the time of treatment must be stored under very strict aseptic conditions for no longer than 24 hours.

3.2.Specific measures

3.2.1. Tracheobronchial suction

3.2.1.1.   Purpose and indications

The aim of tracheobronchial suctioning is to reduce airway congestion in intubated or tracheostomised patients in order to keep their airways clear. This repeated suctioning must be aseptic to avoid inoculating germs, which can cause airway infection.

The indications for tracheobronchial aspiration are :

- bronchial hypersecretion ;
- airway obstruction ;
- presence of secretions in ventilation devices ;
- cough, patient off ventilator ;
- agitation, desaturation.

3.2.1.2.   Equipment and products required

- Vacuum source with pressure gauge ;
- A closed suction system comprising a suction jar and a disposable collection bag;
- Two single-use tubes: one connecting the jar to the vacuum source, the other connecting the jar to the patient;
- A single-use "stop-vacuum" valve;
- Disposable suction catheters;
- A bottle of sterile water or physiological serum;
- A decontamination system for suction lines;
- Non-sterile single-use gloves, gowns and masks;
- Sterile compresses ;
- Antiseptic solution (polyvidone iodine such as Betadine® 10%);

- Hydro-alcoholic solution or antiseptic soap ;
- Bag for infectious risk healthcare waste (yellow).

3.2.1.3.   Technical

- Before handling anything, always disinfect your hands by washing them hygienically or rubbing them with a hydro-alcoholic solution;
- Wearing a gown and mask;
- If necessary, disable the respirator alarm;
- Putting on gloves;
- Open packaging: probe and compresses;
- Soak the compresses in antiseptic ;
- Fit the packaged suction probe to the vacuum stop;
- Remove the packaging and pick up the probe;
- Open the Mount connector with the antiseptic-soaked compress;
- Insert the probe without aspirating into the Mount connection with the vacuum stop open to avoid causing microulcerations;
- Reassemble the probe using suction with a vacuum stop;
- If new suction is required: do not completely remove the probe from the Mount connector and reinsert it with the vacuum stop open;
- Close the Mount connector with a compress soaked in antiseptic;
- Adapt the vacuum stop probe;
- Dispose of the catheter and compresses in the infectious risk waste bag;
- Rinse the suction system: fit the vacuum stop to the decontamination system or to the bottle of sterile water and suction until the secretions in the tube have been evacuated;
- Leave the vacuum stop in place on the decontamination system or the sterile water bottle;
- Dispose of gloves, mask and gown in the infectious waste bag;
- If necessary, reactivate the ventilator alarm;
- Disinfect your hands by washing them hygienically or rubbing them with a hydro-alcoholic solution.

The sterile water bottle is changed at least once every 24 hours. The suction bag is changed if it is full, or systematically after 7 days' use with the suction tube (jar/patient) and the vacuum stop.

3.2.2. Nasopharyngeal suction

3.2.2.1.   Purpose and indications

The aim of nasopharyngeal suctioning is to relieve congestion in a patient's airways, keeping the nasal and pharyngeal cavities clean by repeated suctioning through a dedicated tube.

3.2.2.2. Equipment and products required

The equipment needed is identical to that required for tracheobronchial suctioning.

3.2.2.3. Technical

• Before handling anything, always disinfect your hands by washing them hygienically or rubbing them with a hydro-alcoholic solution;
• Wearing a gown and mask;
• If necessary, disable the respirator alarm;
• Putting on gloves;
• Open packaging: probe and compresses;
• Soak the compresses in antiseptic ;
• Fit the packaged suction probe to the vacuum stop;
• Remove the packaging and pick up the probe;
• Open the Mount connector with the antiseptic-soaked compress;
• Introduce the probe without aspirating with the vacuum stop open to avoid causing microulcerations;
• Reassemble the probe by suction with vacuum stop;
• Suck into the mouth and then the nose;
• Rinse the suction system: fit the vacuum stop to the decontamination system or to the bottle of sterile water and suction until the secretions in the tube have been evacuated;
• Leave the vacuum stop in place on the decontamination system or the sterile water bottle;
• Dispose of gloves, mask and overblouse in the infectious risk waste bag;
• If necessary, reactivate the ventilator alarm;
• Disinfect your hands by washing them hygienically or rubbing them with a hydro-alcoholic solution.

Use a new probe for each aspiration sequence.

3.2.3. Aerosoltherapy

3.2.3.1. Purpose and indications

This technique involves administering a medicinal solution into the airways by nebulisation with a gas. It is a nursing procedure administered on medical prescription.

3.2.3.2. Materials and products required

• Pressure generator ;
• Oxygen wall socket with pressure gauge and connection or an electric compressor;
• Sprayer ;
• Single-dose physiological serum ;

- Sterile sampling equipment for the extemporaneous preparation of aerosol solution;
- Sterile compresses ;
- Bottle of sterile water (for rinsing the nebuliser) ;
- Disposable tissues and spittoons;
- Infectious risk waste bags.

3.2.3.3.   Technical

- Plan the treatment away from meals and samples and before the kinesitherapy session;
- Disinfect hands by washing hygienically or rubbing with a hydro-alcoholic solution;
- Prepare the nebuliser: aseptically remove the drug and mix it with the solvent or physiological serum;
- Place the patient in a semi-seated position;
- Blow your nose and spit;
- Ask the patient to inhale deeply through the nose and exhale deeply through the mouth during the session;
- Plug the device, check that it works and adjust to 6 litres of oxygen per minute;
- Make sure the mask seals tightly around the face;
- Stop the aerosol 15 minutes later and empty the remaining solution;
- Disinfect your hands by washing them hygienically or rubbing them with a hydro-alcoholic solution.

Use only sterile water, never add water to a previously prepared solution. The nebuliser is rinsed with sterile water and wiped dry after each use, and is changed at least once a week.

3.2.4. Oxygen therapy

3.2.4.1.   Purpose and indications

Oxygen therapy involves introducing oxygen into a patient's tracheobronchial tree to improve the concentration of oxygen in the blood. It is a nursing procedure administered on medical prescription.

Oxygen therapy presents a potential risk of drying out the respiratory system, requiring humidification, and a risk of nosocomial respiratory infections.

It is important to respect the following oxygen flow rates:
- 3 litres/minute for a treatment lasting a few days ;
- 2 litres/minute for long-term treatment.

Humidification is necessary in both cases. For flows < 3 litres/minute maintained for a few days, humidification is not necessary. Use only sterile water for humidification.

3.2.4.2. Materials and products required

- A pressure regulator;
- A closed-system humidifier, if available;
- A bottle of sterile water;
- An oxygen administration system: tube or mask;
- Liquid detergent soap.

It is preferable to use a single-use closed system for humidifying the oxygen, or to disinfect it.

It is recommended to change :

- Nasal probe: once a day for continuous use and after each use for discontinuous use;
- Mask: once a week.

3.2.4.3. Technical

- Place the patient in a half-seated position;
- Clearing the upper airways;
- Simple hand washing ;
- Connect the pressure gauge to the wall socket;
- Prepare the humidification system, taking care to use only sterile water and noting the date the system was first used;
- Connect the oxygen tubing to the humidifier;
- Fitting and adapting oxygen administration accessories: mask or tube;
- Adjust the oxygen flow as prescribed;
- Monitor the correct operation of the system and the effectiveness of the treatment (staining of the teguments);
- Record the treatment on the monitoring sheet;
- Do a simple wash.

3.2.5. Inserting and monitoring a nasogastric tube

3.2.5.1. Purpose and indications

The nasogastric tube is a medical device that may be used for therapeutic, diagnostic or nutritional purposes. Inserting a nasogastric tube is an invasive procedure, for which it is essential to take hygiene precautions during insertion and handling, and to introduce monitoring to prevent any risk of infection or secondary complications. Fitting the catheter is a nursing procedure carried out on medical prescription. The nurse is responsible for monitoring the device.

3.2.5.2. Materials and products required

- Adapted probe ;
- Lubricant (Vaseline oil, water) ;
- Glass of water ;
- Feeding syringe ;

- Single-use paper towel ;
- Bean ;
- Adhesive (sometimes nasal fixation with a suture can be chosen);
- Stethoscope ;
- Non-sterile compresses;
- Single-use non-sterile gloves ;
- Bag for infectious risk healthcare waste ;
- Probe shutter ;
- For suction, add a suction jar and a vacuum gauge or a collection bag;
- For a gastric fluid sample, add: a labelled jar for the sample and sterile compresses.

Plastic-coated polyvinyl chloride or PVC probes are used for short surveys (3 to 4 days) and mainly for sampling. Polyurethane probes are used for longer surveys.

Enteral feeding tubes are generally small-bore. Tubes for gastro-duodenal aspirations can be single- or double-channel. The double channel allows gentle aspiration by allowing air to enter the cavity.

This preserves the gastric mucosa. Large-calibre probes are reserved for occlusions or digestive bleeding. All probes are fitted with graduation markers and are radio-opaque.

The lubricant should not be silicone-based if the probe is silicone. Water seems to be the best lubricant.

3.2.5.3.   Technical

- Outside the emergency context, the patient must be fasting or at least four to six hours after the last meal;
- Place the patient in a semi-seated position;
- Disinfect hands by washing hygienically or rubbing with a hydro-alcoholic solution;
- Place the patient in a semi-seated position with the neck flexed;
- Determine the length of the probe d introduce: measure the distance from the nose to the xiphoid appendage, passing through the ear, and mark an indelible reference point;
- Put on disposable gloves;
- Lubricate the probe with a compress;
- Introduce the probe into the nostril and push it slowly without forcing until it reaches the glottis ;
- Encourage the patient to swallow (1 glass of water may help);
- Push the probe to the desired mark;
- Check that the tube is in the stomach (aspirate the gastric contents, inject air

into the tube and listen with the stethoscope placed in the epigastric cavity: a characteristic aerial noise should be heard). If in doubt, repeat the procedure and/or ask for a follow-up X-ray;
- Fix the probe with adhesive;
- Block the catheter or implement the prescription: suction or nutrition;
- Note the date of application on the treatment form.

3.2.5.4.   Monitoring and hygiene care

Monitoring

The position of the probe is checked daily. This is done by looking for the marker initially determined and keeping it in the correct position, completed by checking that the tube is correctly positioned in the stomach by injecting air and listening with the stethoscope. This operation should be repeated systematically whenever the tube is used for nutritional, therapeutic or water administration purposes.

The permeability of the catheter must be checked to prevent any obstruction. The catheter should always be rinsed with between 30 and 50 ml of water after use.

If there is an obstruction, it can be cleared by rinsing with pressurised water using a syringe, but be careful: the catheter may be displaced, and an X-ray may be necessary before clearing the obstruction in this situation. Caution: never undertake a deobstruction manoeuvre with a chuck.

To prevent gastro-resophageal reflux, the patient should be placed in a semi-seated position whenever the tube is used.

It is also essential to monitor the integrity of the nasal and oral mucosa. We watch for the appearance of ulceration and necrosis. Prevention is ensured by daily local hygiene care.

Hygiene care

Mouth care: performed at least twice a day; if the patient is sufficiently cooperative, mouthwash may be preferable.

Nose care: Change the adhesive daily, change the point of support of the probe to prevent the appearance of a nasal ulcer. Regularly instill physiological saline into the nostrils.

XII- PREVENTION OF VENOUS CATHETER-RELATED INFECTIONS

1. INTRODUCTION

Bacteremia/septicemia and catheter infections account for almost 7% of nosocomial infections in developed countries. The frequency of these infections remains high in certain high-risk departments such as intensive care, oncology and neonatology. The main risk factor for these infections, which are often very serious, is the use of a venous catheter, whether central or peripheral.

Venous catheterisation involves introducing a short or long, single- or multi-lumen catheter into the venous system, either transcutaneously or surgically. Venous catheterisation involves :

- *or the superficial veins:* this is peripheral venous catheterisation;
- *or the deep venous trunks: this is* the central venous catheter.

The catheter creates a breach in the skin surface, providing an entry point for bacterial invasion.

2. PREVENTION OF INFECTIONS RELATED TO PERIPHERAL VENOUS CATHETERS

2.1. Definition and indications

Peripheral venous catheterisation involves inserting a short catheter transcutaneously into the venous system. Inserting a short peripheral venous catheter is a nursing procedure, on medical prescription.

The peripheral venous line must be used for clearly defined therapeutic or diagnostic indications: rehydration, drug treatment or transfusion.

The indications for these invasive devices must be kept to a minimum, weighing up the risks against the expected benefits in each case.

2.2. Integration sites

Venous infusion sites in the lower limbs should be avoided. Preference should be given to the forearm and hand, avoiding the folds (elbow and wrist).

Do not sting:

- on the side with an arteriovenous fistula ;
- on the side with an orthopaedic or vascular prosthesis ;
- on the side of lymph node or axillary removal or radiotherapy;
- the hemiplegic side ;
- limbs with skin lesions or an infectious site close to the insertion site.

The insertion site is charged systematically every 72 a 96 hours.

2.3. Materials and products required
- Gueridon or tray for individual care;
- Bean and/or bag a waste a infectious risk (yellow) ;
- Collector a sharps waste ;
- Clean and disinfect tourniquet between each patient;
- Single-use non-sterile gloves;
- Clippers or depilatory cream if there is significant pilosity which may prevent the dressing from holding in place;
- Foaming antiseptic solution and antiseptic from the same range (polyvidone iodine such as Betadine® or its equivalent);
- Sterile water or physiological serum;
- Sterile compresses ;
- Short venous catheters (several sizes available);
- Sterile plasters ;
- Infusion bottle with purged tubing ;
- Extender fitted with a a 3-way tap.

Metal needles and polyurethane and Teflon catheters appear to be less irritating than PVC catheters.

2.4. Catheter insertion
- Simply wash your hands or rub them with a hydroalcoholic solution;
- Locate the vein to be catheterised using a tourniquet;
- Prepare the equipment needed for the procedure on a work surface;
- Disinfect hands by washing hygienically or by rubbing with a hydro-alcoholic solution and put on disposable gloves;
- 4-step skin antisepsis :
1. *Detersion:* Cleanse the skin with the foaming antiseptic solution;
2. *Ringing :* Rinse with sterile water;
3. *Drying:* Dry with sterile compresses;
4. *Antisepsis:* Apply the antiseptic solution liberally from the insertion site using sterile compresses and leave for one minute.
- Insert the catheter, dispose of the mandrel in the sharps waste collector as close as possible to the procedure and connect the infusion using an extension lead fitted with a 3-way stopcock;
- Fix the catheter correctly with a sterile plaster after checking for reflux and cover with an occlusive dressing, leaving the 3-way valve outside;
- Note the date of insertion on the dressing and on the patient record, specifying the location of the catheter;
- Dispose of the equipment in accordance with the procedure for disposing of healthcare waste and disinfect your hands by washing them hygienically or

rubbing them with hydro-alcoholic solutions.

2.5. Handling the catheter

• Before handling anything, always disinfect your hands by washing them hygienically or rubbing them with a hydro-alcoholic solution;

• Use sterile compresses soaked in antiseptic (polyvidone-iodine such as Betadine® or its equivalent) for the openings in the venous line and change the disposable plugs after each use;

• The interval for changing infusion tubing and accessories (valves, infusion manifold) is 72 to 96 hours, except in the case of transfusion or lipid infusion, when they are changed immediately after the products have been infused;

• The extension tube attached to the catheter is considered to be part of the catheter and not part of the venous line: it is therefore not affected by the rate at which the tubing is changed. It is changed at the same time as the catheter;

• There is no need to change the dressing periodically, whatever its type, as long as it remains occlusive and is not soiled;

• Aseptic and extemporaneous preparation of infusion solutions;

• Rinse the catheter with physiological serum after each discontinuous infusion (parenteral nutrition, antibiotic therapy);

• In the case of a catheter with a mouth, it is preferable to change the site rather than forcibly unblocking the catheter, as there is a risk of embolism.

2.6. Catheter removal

The catheter is removed:

• As soon as it is no longer necessary;

• After 72 to 96 hours (increased risk of infection after this time). If it is necessary to preserve the venous capital, this time may be extended, subject to rigorous monitoring.

• Imperatively in case of local intolerance reaction, suspicion of phlebitis and local or general infectious clinical signs;

• When the catheter is blocked.

In all cases, it is essential to note the date of removal, specifying the reason if it corresponds to a problem encountered.

3. PREVENTION OF INFECTIONS RELATED TO CENTRAL VENOUS CATHETERS

3.1. Definition and indications

Central venous catheterisation involves inserting a long catheter into the venous system, giving access to the right atrium/cavernous system junction. The catheter is implanted percutaneously or surgically. Inserting a central venous catheter is a medical procedure. The nurse is responsible for maintenance, monitoring and follow-up.

The indications for central venous catheterisation must be kept to a minimum. This invasive device is used in cases of :
- alteration of peripheral venous capital ;
- intravenous administration of products that are aggressive to the veins;
- administration of hypertonic solutions ;
- heavy or iterative chemotherapy ;
- major transfusion of blood or blood derivatives.

3.2. Integration sites

Except in emergency situations, the superior vena cava is preferred. Any catheter inserted in an emergency should be changed as soon as the patient's situation has stabilised, except when the required aseptic conditions have been met.

3.3. Materials and products required

- Gueridon or tray for individual care;
- Bean and/or bag of infectious risk waste (yellow) ;
- Sharps waste collector ;
- Bed protector ;
- Sterile surgical gown;
- Sterile drapes ;
- Sterile gloves;
- Clippers or depilatory cream if there is significant pilosity which may prevent the dressing from holding in place;
- Foaming antiseptic solution and antiseptic from the same range (polyvidone iodine such as Betadine® or its equivalent);
- Sterile water or physiological serum;
- Sterile compresses ;
- Long vein catheters ;
- Xylocaine 2% non-adrenaline, 10 cc syringe, trocar and intramuscular needle, tap ramp, extension tube;
- Sterile plasters ;
- Infusion bottle with purged tubing ;
- Straight or curved needle thread with needle holder, sterile scissors or scalpel blade.

The catheter used must be chosen according to its intended use and the foreseeable duration of its use: central catheters made of polyurethane or silicone elastomer are less thrombogenic and less susceptible to bacterial adhesion than those made of PVC or Teflon. However, their use is only clinically justified for prolonged use (more than 10 days).

Multiple lumen catheters present a slightly higher risk of infection than single lumen catheters. Their use should therefore be restricted to intensive care and resuscitation units. In practice, the main risk factor appears to be the frequency with which the venous line is manipulated and the absence of a closed system, due to the aseptic errors that may be associated with all these manoeuvres.

Implantable sites, subcutaneous collagen and silver sleeves and catheters impregnated with antibacterial agents have not yet been formally proven to be effective in preventing the development of infections.

Continuous or discontinuous heparinisation has not proved its worth.

3.4. Catheter insertion

A central catheter must be inserted under conditions of surgical asepsis, by an experienced operator and a trained team, with the number of personnel present in the vicinity of the patient limited to the minimum required. The instructions are as follows:

- The operator and his assistant must perform surgical hand washing or hand disinfection by surgical friction using hydro-alcoholic solutions;
- Operators must be dressed in a cap, mask, gown and sterile gloves;
- Patients can wear a mask depending on their respiratory condition;
- If the hair is a problem for the bandage, remove it using clippers or depilatory cream to avoid micro-cuts;
- The nurse performs surgical-level skin antisepsis in 5 steps:

1. *Detersion:* Cleanse the skin with the foaming antiseptic solution;
2. *Ringing :* Rinse with sterile water;
3. *Drying:* Dry with sterile compresses;
4. *1ère Antisepsis:* Apply the antiseptic solution in a centrifugal manner starting from the insertion site using sterile compresses and leave to dry;
5. *2eme Antisepsis:* leave to dry.

- The operating area is set up with wide sterile drapes;
- The catheter must be firmly attached to the skin and checked regularly;
- The surgeon must apply an occlusive dressing covering the puncture site and the catheter hub and note the date of insertion on a document reserved for this purpose;
- X-rays should be taken after insertion to check the catheter path;

3.5. Handling the catheter

As with any venous (or arterial) line, handling must be rigorously aseptic and kept to a minimum. Other recommendations are as follows:

- Before handling anything, always disinfect your hands by washing them hygienically or rubbing them with a hydro-alcoholic solution;
- The infusion rails are fixed to a support as far away from the patient as possible;

- The closed system must be respected;
- Tubes, taps and stoppers are handled using a compress soaked in an antiseptic (polyvidone-iodine such as Betadine® or its equivalent);
- The plugs are changed each time they are handled;
- Tubing should be changed every 72 to 96 hours, except when administering labile blood products or lipid emulsions, when tubing should be changed after each passage;
- The extension connected directly to the catheter is not changed during the entire catheter insertion period. It is considered to be integrated into the catheter;
- In the absence of soiling or detachment, the dressing re-dressing interval can be extended to 5 to 7 days, but any soiled or non-occlusive dressing must be changed without delay.

3.6. Catheter removal

Removal is prescribed by a doctor. It is systematic:
- As soon as it is no longer essential;
- If it is blocked ;
- If there are signs of infection (local inflammation, chills, febrile spikes).

Removal is an aseptic procedure, and a sterile dressing is applied for at least 24 hours.

References

1- Guide technique d'hygiène hospitaliere - Author GIRARD, R; MONNET, D; -FABRY J.

2- Manuel d'hygiène a l'usage des dtaɔlissements hospitaliers - Dr A. Atif , Abdeljalil Bezzaoucha.

3- Rdfdrentiel mdtier : Spdcialistes er. Hygiene, Prevention, Controle de l'Infection en milieu de soins - March 2018.

4- Improving the identification process for air and surface samples in LIMS for hospital hygiene matrices J Bailly - 2019 - hal.univ-lorraine.fr

5- L'Hygiene Hospitaliere: Que Do-On En Attendre Aujourd'Hui JJ Haxhe - Acta Clinica Belgica, 1982 - Taylor & Francis

6- Hospital Hygiene-N Hygis - 1998 - books.google.com

7- conceptual bases and fields of hospital hygiene kammoun - hospital hygiene: concepts, fields and ..., 2008 - sotugeres.org

8- Hospital hygiene and the prevention of healthcare-associated infections -O Meunier - L'Aide-Soignante, 2018 - Elsevier

9- Hand hygiene and nosocomial infections in intensive care -C Saint Sorny, A Duquesne. N Boumrar, M Hulin. - Annales Frangaises d' .., 2014 - Elsevier

10- Nosocomial infections of bacterial origin, what the dispensing pharmacist needs to know -A Albrecht - 2015 - hal.univ-lorraine.f-.

11- Prevention of Nosocomial Infections in Hospitals -A Moumene - dspace.univ-tlemcen.dz

12- Hospital hygiene manual for use in hospitals -M. Atif, A.Bezzaoucha

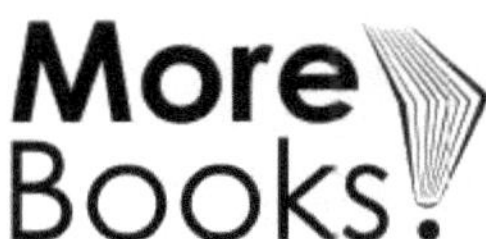

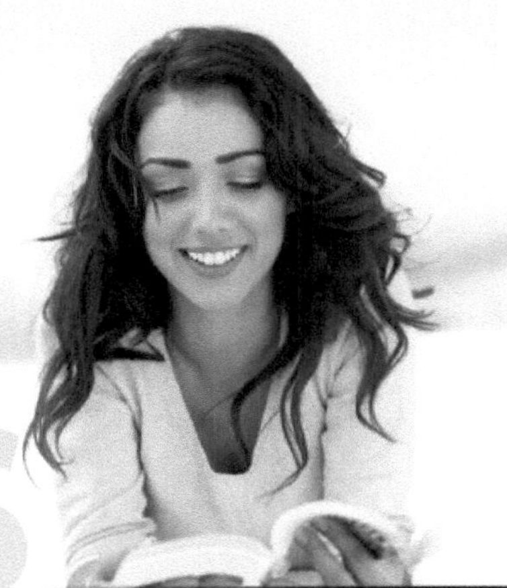

I want morebooks!

Buy your books fast and straightforward online - at one of world's fastest growing online book stores! Environmentally sound due to Print-on-Demand technologies.

Buy your books online at
www.morebooks.shop

Kaufen Sie Ihre Bücher schnell und unkompliziert online – auf einer der am schnellsten wachsenden Buchhandelsplattformen weltweit! Dank Print-On-Demand umwelt- und ressourcenschonend produziert.

Bücher schneller online kaufen
www.morebooks.shop

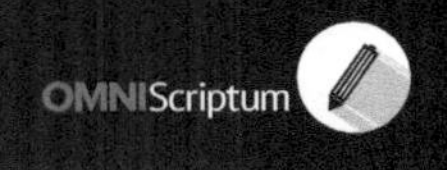